Digital Health

Editors

DIPTI ITCHHAPORIA
RAGAVENDRA R. BALIGA

HEART FAILURE CLINICS

www.heartfailure.theclinics.com

Consulting Editor
EDUARDO BOSSONE

Founding Editor
JAGAT NARULA

April 2022 • Volume 18 • Number 2

ELSEVIER

1600 John F. Kennedy Boulevard • Suite 1800 • Philadelphia, Pennsylvania, 19103-2899

http://www.theclinics.com

HEART FAILURE CLINICS Volume 18, Number 2
April 2022 ISSN 1551-7136, ISBN-13: 978-0-323-92019-3

Editor: Joanna Collett
Developmental Editor: Jessica Cañaberal

Heart Failure Clinics (ISSN 1551-7136) is published quarterly by Elsevier Inc., 360 Park Avenue South, New York, NY 10010-1710. Months of publication are January, April, July, and October. Business and editorial offices: 1600 John F. Kennedy Boulevard, Suite 1800, Philadelphia, PA 19103-2899. Periodicals postage paid at New York, NY, and additional mailing offices. Subscription prices are USD 277.00 per year for US individuals, USD 681.00 per year for US institutions, USD 100.00 per year for US students and residents, USD 300.00 per year for Canadian individuals, USD 701.00 per year for Canadian institutions, USD 315.00 per year for international individuals, USD 701.00 per year for international institutions, and USD 100.00 per year for Canadian and foreign students/residents. To receive student and resident rate, orders must be accompanied by name of affiliated institution, date of term, and the *signature* of program/residency coordinator on institution letterhead. Orders will be billed at individual rate until proof of status is received. Foreign air speed delivery is included in all *Clinics* subscription prices. All prices are subject to change without notice. **POSTMASTER:** Send address changes to *Heart Failure Clinics*, Elsevier Health Sciences Division, Subscription Customer Service, 3251 Riverport Lane, Maryland Heights, MO 63043. **Customer Service: 1-800-654-2452 (US and Canada). From outside of the US and Canada, call 314-447-8871. Fax: 314-447-8029. For print support, E-mail: JournalsCustomerService-usa@elsevier.com. For online support, E-mail: JournalsOnlineSupport-usa@elsevier.com.**

Reprints. For copies of 100 or more of articles in this publication, please contact the Commercial Reprints Department, Elsevier Inc., 360 Park Avenue South, New York, NY 10010-1710. Tel.: 212-633-3874; Fax: 212-633-3820; E-mail: reprints@elsevier.com.

Heart Failure Clinics is covered in *MEDLINE/PubMed (Index Medicus)*.

Contributors

CONSULTING EDITOR

EDUARDO BOSSONE, MD, PhD, FCCP, FESC, FACC
Director, Division of Cardiology, AORN Antonio Cardarelli Hospital, Naples, Italy

EDITORS

DIPTI ITCHHAPORIA, MD, FACC, FAHA, FESC
President, American College of Cardiology, Eric and Sheila Samson Endowed Chair of Cardiovascular Health, Director of Disease Management, Hoag Memorial Hospital Presbyterian, Newport Beach, California, USA; Associate Clinical Professor, University of California, Irvine, Irvine, California, USA

RAGAVENDRA R. BALIGA, MD, MBA, FACP, FRCP, FACC
Inaugural Director, Cardio-Oncology Center of Excellence, Professor of Internal Medicine, The Ohio State University Wexner Medical Center, Columbus, Ohio, USA

AUTHORS

FARAZ S. AHMAD, MD, MS
Assistant Professor of Medicine, Division of Cardiology, Departments of Medicine and Preventive Medicine, Northwestern University Feinberg School of Medicine, Bluhm Cardiovascular Institute Center for Artificial Intelligence, Northwestern Medicine, Chicago, Illinois, USA

SANJEEV P. BHAVNANI, MD, FACC
Section of Advanced Heart Failure, Division of Cardiology, Principal Investigator Healthcare Innovation and Practice Transformation Laboratory, Scripps Research Foundation, La Jolla, California, USA

BIYKEM BOZKURT, MD, PhD
Michael E. DeBakey VA Medical Center, Winters Center for Heart Failure Research, Cardiovascular Research Institute, Baylor College of Medicine, Houston, Texas, USA

KHADIJAH BREATHETT, MD, MS
Division of Cardiovascular Medicine, Sarver Heart Center, University of Arizona, Tucson, Arizona, USA

LAPRINCESS C. BREWER, MD, MPH
Division of Preventive Cardiology, Department of Cardiovascular Medicine, Mayo Clinic College of Medicine, Rochester, Minnesota, USA

MELVIN R. ECHOLS, MD
Division of Cardiovascular Medicine, Morehouse School of Medicine, Atlanta, Georgia, USA

KANWAL M. FAROOQI, MD
Department of Pediatrics, Division of Cardiology, Columbia University Irving Medical Center, New York, New York, USA

SAVITRI FEDSON, MD, MA
Michael E. DeBakey VA Medical Center, Center for Medical Ethics and Health Policy, Baylor College of Medicine, Houston, Texas, USA; Winters Center for Heart Failure Research

GAVIN W. HICKEY, MD
Division of Cardiology, University of Pittsburgh School of Medicine, Pittsburgh, Pennsylvania, USA

JAMES L. JANUZZI Jr. MD
Department of Medicine, Division of Cardiology, Massachusetts General Hospital, Department of Medicine, Division of Cardiology, Harvard Medical School, Baim Institute for Clinical Research, Boston, Massachusetts, USA

AMBER E. JOHNSON, MD, MS, MBA
University of Pittsburgh School of Medicine Heart and Vascular Institute, Veterans Affairs Pittsburgh Health System, Pittsburgh, Pennsylvania, USA

ULRICH P. JORDE, MD
Department of Internal Medicine, Division of Cardiology, Montefiore Medical Center, Albert Einstein College of Medicine, Bronx, New York, USA

NOBUYUKI KAGIYAMA, MD, PhD
Departments of Digital Health and Telemedicine R&D, and Cardiovascular Biology and Medicine, Juntendo University, Tokyo, Japan

MANREET K. KANWAR, MD
Cardiovascular Institute, Allegheny Health Network, Pittsburgh, Pennsylvania, USA

DAVID P. KAO, MD
Medical Director, Colorado Center for Personalized Medicine, University of Colorado School of Medicine, Physician Informaticist, UC Health, Aurora, Colorado, USA

ROLA KHEDRAKI, MD
Section of Advanced Heart Failure, Division of Cardiovascular Medicine, Scripps Clinic, Prebys Cardiovascular Institute, La Jolla, California, USA

MATTHEW M. LANDER, MD
Cardiovascular Institute, Allegheny Health Network, Pittsburgh, Pennsylvania, USA

SONG LI, MD
Division of Cardiology, University of Washington, Seattle, Washington, USA

FRANCISCO LOPEZ-JIMENEZ, MD, MS, MBA
Consultant, Department of Cardiovascular Medicine, Mayo Clinic, Professor of Medicine, Mayo Medical School, Rochester, Minnesota, USA

YUAN LUO, PhD
Associate Professor, Department of Preventive Medicine, Northwestern University Feinberg School of Medicine, Bluhm Cardiovascular Institute Center for Artificial Intelligence, Northwestern Medicine, Chicago, Illinois, USA

SULA MAZIMBA, MD, MPH
Division of Cardiovascular Medicine, University of Virginia, Charlottesville, Virginia, USA

SAM A. MICHELHAUGH, BA
Georgetown University School of Medicine, Washington, DC, USA

JAI KUMAR NAHAR, MD, MBA
Attending, Division of Cardiology, Children's National Heart Institute, Children's National Hospital, Clinical Associate Professor of Pediatrics, George Washington University School of Medicine and Health Sciences, Washington, DC, USA

PARTHO P. SENGUPTA, MD, DM
Division of Cardiovascular Diseases, Rutgers Robert Wood Johnson Medical School, New Brunswick, New Jersey, USA

RASHMEE U. SHAH, MD, MS
Division of Cardiovascular Medicine, University of Utah, Salt Lake City, Utah, USA

SANJIV J. SHAH, MD
Stone Professor of Medicine, Division of Cardiology, Department of Medicine, Director, Center for Deep Phenotyping and Precision Therapeutics, Institute for Augmented Intelligence in Medicine, Northwestern University Feinberg School of Medicine, Director of Research, Bluhm Cardiovascular Institute Center for Artificial Intelligence, Northwestern Medicine, Chicago, Illinois, USA

JENNIFER SMERLING, MD
Department of Pediatrics, Division of
Cardiology, Columbia University Irving Medical
Center, New York, New York, USA

AJAY V. SRIVASTAVA, MD
Section of Advanced Heart Failure, Division of
Cardiovascular Medicine, Scripps Clinic,
Prebys Cardiovascular Institute, La Jolla,
California, USA

JAMES D. THOMAS, MD
Professor of Medicine, Division of Cardiology,
Department of Medicine, Northwestern
University Feinberg School of Medicine, Bluhm

Cardiovascular Institute Center for Artificial
Intelligence, Northwestern Medicine, Chicago,
Illinois, USA

MÁRTON TOKODI, MD, PhD
Heart and Vascular Center, Semmelweis
University, Budapest, Hungary

RAMSEY M. WEHBE, MD, MSAI
Fellow, Advanced Heart Failure and Transplant
Cardiology, Division of Cardiology, Department
of Medicine, Northwestern University Feinberg
School of Medicine, Bluhm Cardiovascular
Institute Center for Artificial Intelligence,
Northwestern Medicine, Chicago, Illinois, USA

Contents

Increasing the global adoption of electronic health records (EHRs) is transforming the delivery of clinical care. EHRs offer tools that are useful in the care of heart failure ranging from individualized risk stratification and decision support to population management. EHR tools can be combined to target specific areas of need such as the standardization of care, improved quality of care, and resource management. Leveraging EHR functionality has been shown to improve select outcomes including guideline-based therapies, reduction in adverse clinical outcomes, and improved cost-efficiency. Central to success is participation by clinicians and patients in the design and feedback of EHR tools.

Telehealth presents opportunities for enhanced care and benefits to patients with heart failure. As technology develops, telehealth is increasingly being integrated into the standard care of heart failure. Telehealth can help enhance timely access and follow-up, facilitate care coordination for diagnostic and management strategies, individualize management, increase opportunities for multidisciplinary care, help implement complementary management strategies, and improve outcomes. Telehealth commonly includes clinician-to-clinician communication; patient interaction with mobile health technologies including remote monitoring, and clinician-to-patient interaction modalities. Despite all the potential benefits of expanded access, telehealth may have limitations especially for vulnerable populations, who are at risk for less access to telehealth modalities and infrastructure. Clinicians and health networks should examine strategies to incorporate telehealth in the management of patients with heart failure. Health care systems should invest in technologies and provide equipment and connectivity to ensure that telehealth does not widen health disparities.

Consider these 2 scenarios: Two individuals with heart failure (HF) have recently established with your clinic and followed for medical management and risk stratification. One is a 62-year-old man with nonischemic cardiomyopathy due to viral myocarditis, an ejection fraction (EF) of 40%, occasional rate-limiting dyspnea, and comorbidities of atrial fibrillation and hypertension. The other is a 75-year-old woman with ischemic cardiomyopathy, an EF of 35%, a prior hospitalization 6 months ago, and persistent symptoms of edema and orthopnea. Both have expressed interest in remote patient monitoring (RPM) with wearable and digital health devices that are commercially available such as a smartwatch-ECG, weight scales, and blood pressure monitoring technologies. While there is enthusiasm from both patients and their clinical teams to engage in a technology-driven approach to care, important questions arise such as "What are the patient requirements for participation in digital health programs?", "Can we anticipate improvements in HF status and lower the risk of future HF events including hospitalizations?", "Do the same type of devices in different patients provide accurate information on physiologic changes toward individualized risk assessments?", and "What are the systematic approaches to integrate digital health workflows and datasets from RPM into clinical HF programs?". Given the importance of such questions, embracing new technologies, as a core competency of a modern health care system requires a deeper understanding of how effective digital health programs can be designed to meet the needs of patients and their clinical teams. In this review, we propose a new framework of "Digital Phenotypes in HF" for how new devices and sensors and their respective datasets can be used to guide treatment and to predict disease trajectories within the heterogeneity of HF. Our objectives are to generate a systematic approach to evaluate digital health devices as they relate to the next phase of RPM in HF, to critically analyze the literature, and to apply the lessons learned from digital devices through present-day, real-world evidence examples.

Machine Learning in Cardiovascular Imaging

Nobuyuki Kagiyama, Márton Tokodi, and Partho P. Sengupta

The number of cardiovascular imaging studies is growing exponentially, and so is the demand to improve the efficacy of the imaging workflow. Over the past decade, studies have demonstrated that machine learning (ML) holds promise to revolutionize cardiovascular research and clinical care. ML may improve several aspects of cardiovascular imaging, such as image acquisition, segmentation, image interpretation, diagnostics, therapy planning, and prognostication. In this review, we discuss the most promising applications of ML in cardiovascular imaging and also highlight the several challenges to its widespread implementation in clinical practice.

Utilizing Artificial Intelligence to Enhance Health Equity Among Patients with Heart Failure

Amber E. Johnson, LaPrincess C. Brewer, Melvin R. Echols, Sula Mazimba, Rashmee U. Shah, and Khadijah Breathett

Patients with heart failure (HF) are heterogeneous with various intrapersonal and interpersonal characteristics contributing to clinical outcomes. Bias, structural racism, and social determinants of health have been implicated in unequal treatment of patients with HF. Through several methodologies, artificial intelligence (AI) can provide models in HF prediction, prognostication, and provision of care, which may help prevent unequal outcomes. This review highlights AI as a strategy to address racial inequalities in HF; discusses key AI definitions within a health equity context; describes the current uses of AI in HF, strengths and harms in using AI; and offers recommendations for future directions.

Using Artificial Intelligence to Better Predict and Develop Biomarkers

Sam A. Michelhaugh and James L. Januzzi Jr.

Advancements in technology have improved biomarker discovery in the field of heart failure (HF). What was once a slow and laborious process has gained efficiency through use of high-throughput omics platforms to phenotype HF at the level of genes, transcripts, proteins, and metabolites. Furthermore, improvements in artificial intelligence (AI) have made the interpretation of large omics data sets easier and improved analysis. Use of omics and AI in biomarker discovery can aid clinicians by identifying markers of risk for developing HF, monitoring care, determining prognosis, and developing druggable targets. Combined, AI has the power to improve HF patient care.

HEART FAILURE CLINICS

SERIES OF RELATED INTEREST

Cardiology Clinics
http://www.cardiology.theclinics.com/
Cardiac Electrophysiology Clinics
https://www.cardiacep.theclinics.com/
Interventional Cardiology Clinics
https://www.interventional.theclinics.com/

THE CLINICS ARE AVAILABLE ONLINE!
Access your subscription at:
www.theclinics.com

Preface

Digital Transformation in Medicine to Enhance Quality of Life, Longevity, and Health Equity

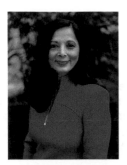
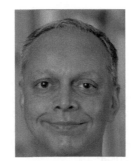
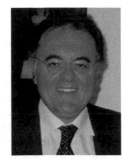

Dipti Itchhaporia, MD, FACC, FAHA, FESC

Ragavendra R. Baliga, MD, MBA, FACP, FRCP, FACC

Eduardo Bossone, MD, PhD, FCCP, FESC, FACC

Editors

Cardiovascular medicine is inherently a "high-tech" profession, with a long history of adopting new technologies to help improve patient outcomes (**Fig. 1**). However, health care delivery to improve efficiency and to optimize health outcomes has not advanced. And while many major sectors of the economy, including finance, transportation, and entertainment, have embraced digital transformation with improved performance metrics, health care has been slower to embrace it.

Successful digital transformation is not just using a new digital technology, such as an app or biosensor, it is the adoption of technologies that make you better at what you do, whether that's improving efficiency or optimizing health and health outcomes.[1]

The American College of Cardiology's innovation program outlines three components of digital transformation that include virtual care, remote patient monitoring, and artificial intelligence (AI)-driven care to help improve patient engagement and satisfaction, clinician efficiency, and satisfaction, as well as health care outcomes.

Technology pervades our everyday lives, and there is no doubt that the future of health care is intimately intertwined with technological advancements. Although AI has existed for over five decades, only recently have we begun to truly realize the potential of its applications, in the form of machine learning (ML), in medical settings. This potential holds the promise of better patient care across all health care institutions by augmenting the work of clinicians. The terms AI, ML, and deep learning are often used interchangeably but are essentially hierarchical. ML methods provide a set of tools to achieve AI and include supervised, unsupervised, and reinforcement learning.[2,3]

In everyday clinical practice, the diagnosis and treatment of cardiovascular disease rely on patient history, physical examination, laboratory data,

Heart Failure Clin 18 (2022) xi–xiii
https://doi.org/10.1016/j.hfc.2022.02.013
1551-7136/22/© 2022 Published by Elsevier Inc.

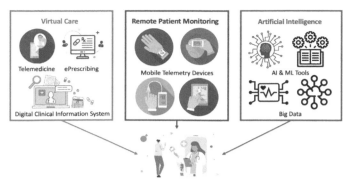

Fig. 1. Digital transformation in health care.

noninvasive imaging diagnostics, and angiography. The introduction of telehealth during the pandemic has further clarified virtual care. Virtual care is much more than telehealth; it should augment or replace what we do now. Ideally it should improve access, efficiency, communication, and the patient experience. Remote patient monitoring with its newer data-rich technologies, including mobile telemetry devices, wearable and implantable recording devices, and other patient-generated health data, should augment virtual care but ultimately requires cardiologists to perform increasingly sophisticated analysis.[4-8]

In the context of this, clinical decision making is a challenging process, with the strain of data overload and the pressure to improve care and translate medical advances and knowledge into an actionable plan. Digital devices using AI tools, specifically ML tools, are poised to potentially extend and augment the effectiveness of the clinician and revolutionize patient care. AI-driven care shows promise for more precise diagnoses, improved image interpretation, streamlined workflows, providing new insights into large data sets that can help with risk prediction, and creation of therapeutic care recommendations.

The explosion of digital technologies that can empower individuals and clinicians to strive for true "health care" rather than sick care is the future of cardiovascular health. While some applications have already found their way into contemporary patient care, we are still in the early days of the digital transformation of health care with digital devices and the AI era in medicine. Despite the popularity of these new technologies, many practitioners lack an understanding of the benefits and pitfalls.

To discuss the promise and tribulations of digital health,[1] including AI and ML, keeping in mind American College of Cardiology guiding principles, we have invited a panel of leading experts in the field to contribute to this issue of *Heart Failure Clinics*. We hope these articles will improve your understanding of this rapidly evolving field and, in turn, allow better care of heart failure patients, improve quality of life, enhancing longevity, and promoting health equity.[9,10]

Dipti Itchhaporia, MD, FACC, FAHA, FESC
American College of Cardiology
Hoag Memorial Hospital Presbyterian
Newport Beach, CA 92663, USA

University of California, Irvine
Irvine, CA 92697, USA

Ragavendra R. Baliga, MD, MBA, FACP, FRCP,
FACC
Division of Cardiology & Cardio-Oncology Center
of Excellence, The Ohio State University Wexner
Medical Center, 452 West 10th Avenue,
Columbus, OH 43210, USA

Eduardo Bossone, MD, PhD, FCCP, FESC, FACC
Division of Cardiology
AORN Antonio Cardarelli Hospital
Naples, Italy

E-mail addresses:
drdipti@yahoo.com (D. Itchhaporia)
rrbaliga@gmail.com (R.R. Baliga)
ebossone@hotmail.com (E. Bossone)

REFERENCES

1. Itchhaporia D. Navigating the path to digital transformation. J Am Coll Cardiol 2021;78(4):412–4.
2. Sardar P, Abbott JD, Kundu A, et al. Impact of artificial intelligence on interventional cardiology: from decision-making aid to advanced interventional procedure assistance. JACC Cardiovasc Interv 2019; 12:1293–303.
3. Petersen SE, Abdulkareem M, Leiner T. Artificial intelligence will transform cardiac imaging-

opportunities and challenges. Front Cardiovasc Med 2019;6:133.

4. Itchhaporia D. Artificial intelligence in cardiology. Trends Cardiovasc Med 2020. https://doi.org/10.1016/j.tcm.2020.11.007.

5. Johnson KW, Soto JT, Glicksberg BS, et al. Artificial intelligence in cardiology. J Am Coll Cardiol 2018;71(23):2668–79.

6. Kuo FC, Mar BG, Lindsley RC, et al. The relative utilities of genome-wide, gene panel, and individual gene sequencing in clinical practice. Blood 2017;130:433–9.

7. Muse ED, Barrett PM, Steinhubl SR, et al. Towards a smart medical home. Lancet 2017;389(10067):358.

8. Steinhubl SR, Muse ED, Topol EJ. The emerging field of mobile health. Sci Transl Med 2015;7(283):283rv3.

9. Itchhaporia D. Population health: intersecting technology, data, health equity to achieve health care transformation. J Am Coll Cardiol 2021;78(15):1569–72.

10. Itchhaporia D. The evolution of the quintuple aim: health equity, health outcomes, and the economy. J Am Coll Cardiol 2021;78(22):2262–4.

Electronic Health Records and Heart Failure

David P. Kao, MD

KEYWORDS

- Heart failure • Electronic health records • Clinical decision support • Predictive analytics
- Care gaps

KEY POINTS

- Electronic health records provide an array of tools including dashboards, analytics, patient portals, and decision support that facilitate the care of patients with congestive heart failure.
- Electronic health record tools can be used for several applications important in the management of heart failure including risk stratification, and care standardization.
- Although mixed, there is evidence that electronic health record tools can be used to improve clinical outcomes, resource utilization, quality of care, and patient satisfaction.
- Electronic health record tools are more useable and useful with clinician design input.

INTRODUCTION

The use of electronic health records (EHRs) is rapidly becoming pervasive in the United States, in part due to requirements established by the Health Information for Economic and Clinical Health (HITECH) Act. Before HITECH, fewer than 10% of physicians used EHRs,[1] whereas following HITECH, nearly 90% of hospitals and clinics have adopted at least a basic EHR.[2] The EHR market globally is now >$30 billion, includes hundreds of countries of all economic status, and ranges from small private practices to national EHR systems. Despite great enthusiasm for the potential of EHRs to improve clinical outcomes, EHR adoption overall has not been associated with improved outcomes and only minimal improvements in care quality in patients with heart failure (HF).[3–5] However, there is evidence that specific EHR-based tools can improve adherence to evidence-based guidelines of HF care, patient self-management, and clinical outcomes.[6] Herein we will review EHR tools useful in managing HF, how they can be used to address specific clinical applications, and evidence supporting their efficacy in improving outcomes (**Fig. 1**). Cited literature is primarily specific to the care of patients with HF given the distinct needs of this population. Whereby no HF-specific data exists, studies involving other diseases or nonselected populations are referenced.

BACKGROUND
EHR components

EHRs are enormously complicated, some costing hundreds of millions of US dollars to implement. Each EHR has specific strengths and weaknesses, which are often based on early priorities and design decisions. EHRs are often described as "digitized medical charts," thereby focusing on clinical documentation. However, many contemporary EHRs are made up of 3 fundamental components: computerized physician order entry (CPOE), clinical documentation and data access, and billing/financial tracking functionality (**Fig. 2**). EHRs increasingly have 2 additional important features: clinical decision support systems (CDSS) and data warehouse capacity. The value of electronic data access in routine clinical care is intuitive and widely apparent, and the addition of data warehouses and health information exchanges is increasing this value further. Billing and financial auditing are crucial capabilities to US institutions in particular and have been the foundation of several commercial EHRs,

University of Colorado School of Medicine, 12700 East 19th Avenue Box B-139, Research Center 2 Room 8005, Aurora, CO 80045, USA
E-mail address: David.Kao@cuanschutz.edu

Heart Failure Clin 18 (2022) 201–211
https://doi.org/10.1016/j.hfc.2021.12.004
1551-7136/22/© 2021 Elsevier Inc. All rights reserved.

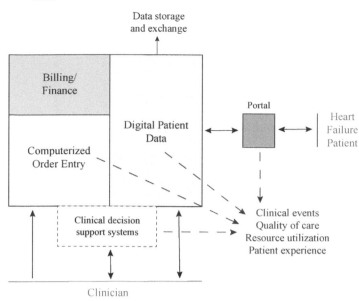

Fig. 1. Electronic health record components and potential benefits to patients with heart failure and their clinicians.

sometimes at the expense of utility and efficiency in clinical care. This discussion will focus on the EHR components that are commonly encountered at the point-of-care and are most useful in the routine clinical care of patients with HF. Knowledge regarding the features discussed should be immediately useful to any HF clinician using EHRs.

Commercial versus free/open-source software

A detailed comparison of the advantages and disadvantages of commercial versus free/open-source software (FOSS) EHRs is beyond the scope of this article. The use of FOSS versus commercial EHRs varies significantly worldwide based on regional constraints and requirements. In general, FOSS EHRs offer dramatically lower implementation costs and greater institution-specific customizability compared with superior development capacity, scalability, technical support including software maintenance, and security of commercial EHRs. Many of the features below, with the possible exception of machine learning (ML) analytics, are available or implementable in most

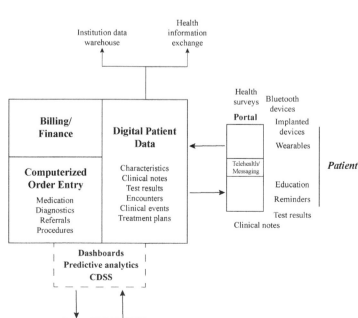

Fig. 2. Electronic health record schematic with major components important for the management of heart failure.

EHRs. This review will not compare components of specific EHR vendors or platforms and will instead discuss features in an EHR-agnostic fashion. Clinicians are encouraged to investigate tools available at their respective institutions.

TOOLS
Dashboards

EHR dashboards summarize patient characteristics, interventions, and other features to monitor and manage groups of patients (**Fig. 3**). Patient cohorts may represent a shared disease condition (eg, HF, diabetes mellitus) or administrative designation (eg, inpatient service, individual clinician panel). A wide range of clinicians (eg, physician, nursing staff, case manager, pharmacist) may access dashboards to monitor clinical status, treatment adherence, health care encounters, test results, and other features, thereby improving efficiency in managing large numbers of patients. For example, HF dashboards can track the use of guideline-directed medical therapy (GDMT) as well as whether the patient is on a target dose of each agent.[7] Many dashboard tools allow a clinician to select a patient of interest to get more detail, open their individual chart, and make management changes as needed. The ability of dashboards to summarize and display diverse data from multiple patients efficiently has led them to become important components of population health management, particularly of chronic diseases.[7,8]

Historically condition-specific dashboards were populated by hand (ie, clinicians select individual patients one by one). More recently, methods for identifying disease cases such as HF are being used to automatically screen patients and even populate dashboards.[9] As the diversity of digital patient data increases, dashboards are increasingly used to aggregate and present data from disparate sources such as remote device measurements, quality of life (QOL) inventories, pharmacy utilization, and test results.[10] Given the complexity and interconnectedness of these new data streams, dashboards will undoubtedly be a critical part of incorporating them into clinician workflows efficiently.

Predictive analytics
There has been a substantial amount of work using EHRs to develop and refine analytical models to guide HF management.[11–13] Methods used to create clinical models from EHR data include regression models, time-to-event or survival models, classification/regression trees, random forest analysis, neural networks, and others, although consistency and completeness of data is a major challenge. Automated HF identification and risk stratification have been the most widely-studied applications although there have been some efforts to predict treatment response.[14] Perhaps the most significant limitation in the use of EHR-based predictive analytics has been the lack of EHR implementation and integration with clinical workflow. Most published EHR-based predictive models were trained on retrospective data extracted from the EHR or accompanying data warehouse, but they are not easily translated to real-time use for a number of reasons. These factors include the complexity of methods, inability of EHRs to execute those methods (eg, ML), uncertain effects on EHR stability, security considerations if using an external server, and operational

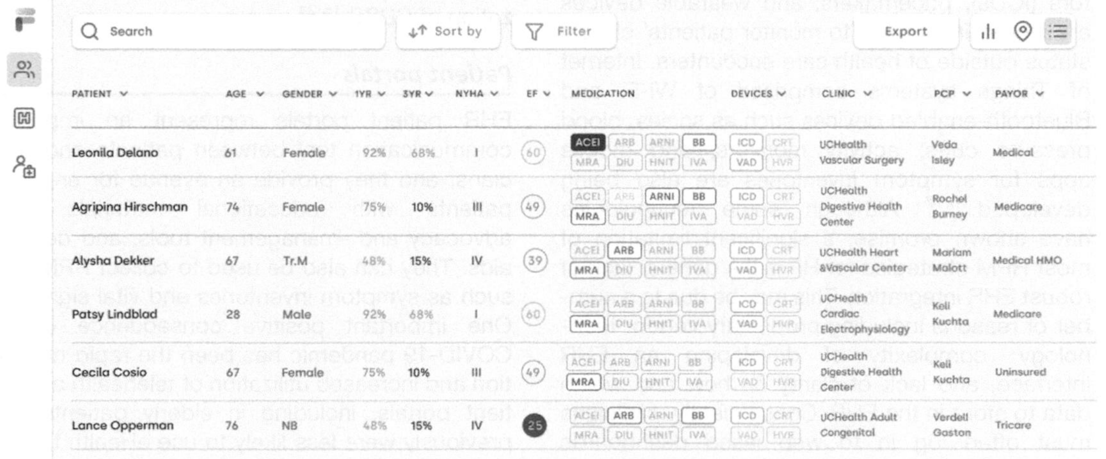

Fig. 3. Patient cohort dashboard example. (*Courtesy of* Codex Health, Inc., Palo Alto, CA)

resources required for implementation. Most importantly, change management in clinician acceptance, behavior, and workflows is critical to translate even high-quality predictions to clinical action.

Standardization frameworks

Applications such as order sets and clinical pathways are used increasingly to promote consistent care across provider groups. When constructed well, order sets and pathways make it easier and faster for clinicians to adhere to recommended management than not to (ie, prespecified orders rather than writing orders from scratch). Order sets and pathways were used long before CPOE was available and today are implemented in largely the same format in EHRs. Added benefits of using EHR-based order sets include the ability to update content and immediately disseminate them in a consistent manner across large health care systems, the potential for modular order sets (eg, components of diabetes mellitus, HF, and chronic obstructive pulmonary disease hospital admission order sets for a patient with multiple comorbidities) and automated presentation of order sets based on the algorithmic ascertainment of disease conditions (eg, suggest a using HF order set for a patient hospitalized with a BNP >150). Order sets and pathways are frequently used to optimize performance metrics as well. Importantly, consideration of human factors elements in the design of HF order sets seems to improve utilization, and clinician participation is strongly encouraged.[15]

Remote patient monitoring

Remote patient monitoring (RPM) using devices such as CardioMEMs, implanted cardiac defibrillators (ICDs), pacemakers, and wearable devices are increasingly used to monitor patients' clinical status outside of health care encounters. Internet of Things systems comprised of Wi-Fi and Bluetooth-enabled devices such as scales, blood pressure cuffs, activity monitors, and mobile apps for symptom inventories are also being developed.[16,17] Although some technologies have shown promise, a significant limitation of most RPM strategies for HF is the general lack of robust EHR integration. This may be due to a number of reasons including proprietary vendor technology, complexity of developing an EHR interface, and lack of clarity on how and which data to store in the EHR. Consequently, clinicians must often log in to web-based dashboards outside of their EHR workflow. Generalizable strategies for generating meaningful signals from remote device data and determining the locus of that processing (ie, internal vs external to the EHR) remain nascent. Workflows to make timely and beneficial use of remotely captured data within health care systems via the EHR are not well-developed. Nevertheless, it is highly likely that the integration of remotely captured data into the EHR will be critical for realizing their full potential.

Clinical decision support

EHR-based CDSS have become essential tools for supporting clinicians during routine care[18] and have shown promise in improving HF outcomes.[19] In reality, all EHR tools described above are forms of clinical decision support. For the purposes of this review, the term CDSS will be used primarily to discuss alert-based functionality. The most commonly encountered CDSS alerts are those identifying drug–drug and drug–allergy interactions, but CDSS are becoming increasingly complex in combination with innovative dashboards, advanced predictive analytics, and care standardization tools. The most general framework of CDSS alerts consists of a logical statement, or "trigger," followed by an alert, either interruptive or passive, to inform the clinician of a recommendation. A simple example is "If the patient's LVEF is less than 40% and they are not on a beta-blocker (BB), then alert the clinician the patient should be on a BB." (**Fig. 4**) Interruptive or active CDS alerts are more effective than passive alerts in modifying clinician behavior including in HF[20,21] but have the greater potential to cause alert fatigue. Careful consideration of details such as clinical impact, alert frequency, recommended action, and workflow disruption is critical to designing effective CDSS.[22,23] As with all tools discussed here, clinician input improves the utilization of CDSS.[15,24]

Patient portals

EHR patient portals represent an important communication tool between patients and clinicians, and they provide an avenue for engaging patients with educational materials, self-advocacy and -management tools, and decision aids. They can also be used to collect RPM data such as symptom inventories and vital signs.[25,26] One important positive consequence of the COVID-19 pandemic has been the rapid maturation and increased utilization of telehealth and patient portals, including in elderly patients who previously were less likely to use eHealth tools.[27] Data regarding the impact of patient portals on clinical outcomes in a general population is limited,

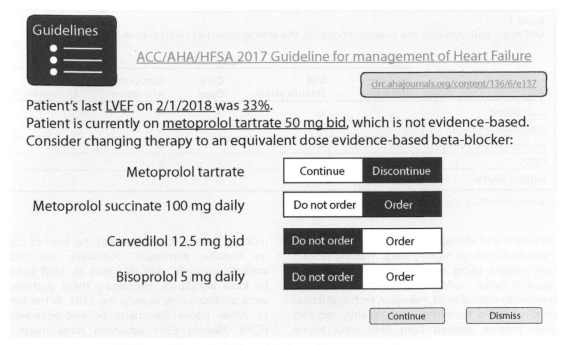

Fig. 4. Generic CDS example – evidence-based beta-blocker adherence.

and a recent Cochrane Review concluded that quality of available results was too low to discern any clinical benefits taken together.[28] However, there is evidence that patient portals may be particularly useful in patients with multiple chronic conditions.[29,30] Availability of a patient's health record via a patient portal can be a valuable tool in the continuity of care compared with traditional requests for their records.

Thus far, sophisticated, multimodal mobile health (mHealth) applications are not widely integrated with EHRs, largely for technical reasons in the variability of interface and EHR specifications between institutions. Efforts are underway to integrate patient-reported outcomes instruments with EHRs,[31] although best practices for using these data have not yet been defined. It is likely that in the future, features of the mHealth applications if not the applications themselves will be integrated with EHR patient portals, but the challenge of EHR interoperability will remain a significant barrier.

APPLICATIONS

Specific clinical tasks are often undertaken using multiple EHR tools (**Table 1**). The choice of each tool is largely determined by the most effective way to impact workflows key to the desired improvements.

Automated diagnosis and risk stratification

Many EHR-based applications rely on identifying patients to whom HF-specific interventions should be applied. Historically, this has been a largely manual process wherein providers or create lists based on chart review or knowledge of the patient. This approach likely resulted in high specificity, but large numbers of undiagnosed patients may have been missed, especially in large health care systems. A variety of strategies have been used to automatically identify patients with HF using EHR data including simple heuristic criteria,[32] natural language processing,[33] and ML models.[34] One application of combined automated HF diagnosis and risk stratification is the identification of patients who may qualify for advanced therapies including implanted devices and transplantation.[35–37] An evolving important application of EHRs is the support of end-of-life care planning, either by the referral or presentation of relevant information such as risk scores and a patient's expressed wishes regarding care goals.[38]

There are many examples of risk stratification models to identify patients with HF and assess their likelihood of adverse clinical events. Rehospitalization within 30 days of discharge is one of the most common endpoints that such models aim to reduce. An increasing proportion of these models are generated and/or validated using EHR data, whereas earlier models relied primarily on

Table 1
EHR tools and common use in applications for the management of heart failure

Tool	Application				
	HF Case Detection	Risk Stratification	Care Gaps	Resource Allocation	Patient Engagement
Dashboard		+	+	+	
Predictive analytics	+	+		+	
Remote monitoring		+		+	+
CDSS	+	+	+	+	
Patient portal			+		+

Abbreviation: CDSS, clinical decision support systems.

derivation and validation using clinical trial, observational cohort, or registry data. Training predictive models using real-world EHR data might result in better performance when finally implemented as clinical tools. However, technical limitations of EHRs have until very recently required even models derived from EHR data to be accessed and return results to clinicians outside of the EHR and normal workflow. The convenience of automated risk stratification can, therefore, increase the likelihood that it will be used in clinical care and leverage more patient data than a clinician typically has time to review, although the presence and accuracy of key variables (eg, New York Heart Association class) can limit practical use.

Care gaps and standardization of management

EHRs seem useful in assessing adherence to HF management guidelines and identifying care gaps,[39] and HF management guidelines can be encoded within EHRs to improve adherence to evidence-based recommendations.[40] Dashboards, predictive analytics, CDSS, and patient portals have all been applied to closing care gaps.[14,25,39,41,42] Although EHR reporting tools and business intelligence are not discussed extensively here, assessment of adherence to care guidelines and quality metrics is a core use of such systems. It should be noted that due to the lack of guidelines and, until recently, effective medications for improving outcomes in HF with preserved ejection fraction, studies and data on EHR-facilitated improvement in care gaps are limited to HF with reduced ejection fraction.

HF-specific care pathways have been demonstrated to improve some HF outcomes, particularly in hospitalized patients.[43–46] These pathways leverage HF-specific order sets but also include guidance regarding decision-making, for example, regarding the level of care on hospital admission. Pathways are often institution-specific and designed by staff based on local workflows. Historically these pathways were available only outside the EHR, in the form of either paper flowcharts or web-accessible PDFs. Recent EHR advances have made it possible to render interactive care pathways for a number of both acute and chronic conditions. In some implementations, patient-specific information is imported automatically, and the clinician can place orders directly from the displayed pathway. Data on interactive EHR-based pathways are limited but do show promise that this may be both an efficient and effective functionality for standardizing care.[47,48]

Resource management

EHR-based predictive analytics may be used in combination with dashboards and CDSS to allocate scarce or costly resources to patients with the highest potential benefit. In doing so, it is possible to coordinate multiple services efficiently in a semiautomated fashion.[49] EHR tools such as order sets and alerts can also be used to optimize the selection of, for example, radiology studies and reduce the use of costly interventions.

OUTCOMES

The above-described applications implemented using EHR tools are also used in several combinations in an effort to improve clinical outcomes, care measures, and system efficiency (**Table 2**). Data regarding the impact of EHRs generally and EHR tools individually is mixed and highly dependent on the institution's clinical actions are taken based on the outputs of these tools. There is marked variation in efficacy between different disease conditions as well. For this discussion, data regarding associations between EHR tools and outcomes

Table 2
EHR tools and impact on heart failure outcomes

	Outcomes			
Tool	Clinical Events	Quality of Care	Cost/ Utilization	Patient Experience
Dashboard	+			
Predictive analytics	+		+	
Remote monitoring				+
CDSS	+	+	+	
Patient portal		+		+

Abbreviation: CDSS, clinical decision support systems.

are presented almost entirely with respect to HF populations.

Care quality

EHR-based interventions have been shown in some studies to increase the use and optimization of certain forms of GDMT for HF, although other analyses have not demonstrated any benefit.[5] The best evidence of EHR efficacy thus far demonstrates increased use of GDMT, in particular BB, angiotensin-converting enzyme inhibitor or angiotensin receptor blocker, mineralocorticoid receptor antagonists, and HF education.[21,41,50,51] EPIC-HF showed that an educational tool regarding GDMT recommendations sent via the EHR patient portal to patients before their clinic visit resulted in greater rates of GDMT intensification than control patients.[25] Intuitively one might expect EHRs to improve rates referral for implanted devices (CRT, LVAD), but data are mixed.[51] The latter may be due to difficulty in encoding the criteria for device therapy referral without resulting in an excess of premature prompts during the optimization of GDMT. However, there are examples of complex patient selection algorithms coupled with targeted CDSS embedded in the EHR that successfully identify and promote referral of appropriate patients to advanced HF services resulting in improved outcomes.[37,52]

Clinical events

Reduction of 30-day hospital readmissions is one of the most widely studied applications of EHR technology in the care of patients with HF. There is some evidence that 30-day readmissions following HF hospitalization may be reduced by using HF dashboards.[53] HF order sets have been associated with increased guideline adherence, decreased length of stay, and all-cause mortality.[54–56] RPM using implanted devices has shown promise in identifying HF decompensation[57,58]

and in some cases, improving HF outcomes such as hospitalization.[59] Availability of RPM data in the EHR is limited, but this is an active area of development and some subset of these data will likely be available in the EHR in the future.

Optimization of predictive analytics identifying patients at high risk for readmission or mortality is a cornerstone of EHR-based efforts to improve patient outcomes. A number of high-performing models predicting hospital readmission have been derived using EHR data, but translating these into reduced HF readmission rates has been complicated (1) implementing models in the EHR and (2) establishing effective accompanying workflows and interventions. Real-time EHR-based predictive analytics that has been combined successfully with clinical interventions have been shown to improve 30-day readmission rates. For example, Amarasingham and colleagues[49] demonstrated that provision of intensive inpatient interventions based on an EHR-based predictive model for 30-day readmission resulted in a reduction in readmission rate from 26.2% to 21.2% (OR 0.73, $P = .01$). Using a different approach, the Stanford HF dashboard leveraged automated HF patient identification tools in combination with a dashboard to improve the utilization of an established readmission reduction program reduced 30-day readmission rates from 14% to 10.1%.[9] Data regarding reduction in clinical events using RPM and EHR patient portals are limited, although there is some evidence that patient engagement with these tools is associated with improved outcomes such as hospital readmission.[60]

Patient experience

Access to EHR data has also been shown to improve engagement, communication with provider team, empowerment, self-education, and self-management behaviors in patients with HF.[61–63] These have been shown in some settings to translate into improved self-care behavior,[63]

QOL,[63] GDMT escalation,[25] and accuracy of EHR data.[64] Electronic capture of patient-reported outcomes such as Kansas City Cardiomyopathy Questionnaire via EHR is also perceived by patients with HF to facilitate communication with their providers and as beneficial to their care.[65]

Cost and resource utilization

General cost savings associated with EHR implementation following the HITECH act is difficult to determine but for Medicare is estimated at $\sim$ \$1 billion/year between 2010 and 2013.[66] With respect to the management of HF, EHRs can reduce costly or unnecessary interventions while increasing the utilization of under-used interventions. EHR-based CDSS has been shown to reduce costs by decreasing redundant or inappropriate testing as well as discouraging the use of potentially harmful medications.[67,68] Access to comprehensive clinical data on presentation to the emergency department can optimize acute care to improve inpatient outcomes including length of hospital stay. As stated earlier, CDSS directed by predictive analytics can also help allocate limited resources and interventions such as multidisciplinary care interventions to high-risk patients.[49] Closing care gaps for invasive therapies can also increase the use of interventions such as ICD, CRT, LVAD, and transplant. Given the high cost of care for the HF population, incremental improvements in efficiency have the potential to result in significant savings on institutional, regional, and national levels.

SUMMARY

EHRs are becoming ubiquitous in modern clinical practice. They offer a wide array of applications that support clinical care including several that have been shown to improve the efficiency and quality of care in patients with HF. EHRs should not be seen as replacements for clinicians and clinical judgment. Clinician participation in design, education in optimal use, and integration of these tools with corresponding workflows can help clinicians to spend less time looking at the EHR and more time caring for the patient.

DISCLOSURE STATEMENT

Dr Kao is supported by National Heart, Lung, and Blood Institute award K08HL125275, as well as L30 HL110124. Dr Kao is an advisor and has received stock options from Codex Health, Inc.

REFERENCES

1. Jha AK, DesRoches CM, Campbell EG, et al. Use of electronic health records in U.S. hospitals. N Engl J Med 2009;360(16):1628–38. https://doi.org/10.1056/NEJMsa0900592.

2. Gold M, McLaughlin C. Assessing HITECH implementation and lessons: 5 years later. Milbank Q 2016;94(3):654–87. https://doi.org/10.1111/1468-0009.12212.

3. Frizzell JD, Liang L, Schulte PJ, et al. Prediction of 30-day all-cause readmissions in patients hospitalized for heart failure: comparison of machine learning and other statistical approaches. JAMA Cardiol 2017;2(2):204–9. https://doi.org/10.1001/jamacardio.2016.3956.

4. Walsh MN, Albert NM, Curtis AB, et al. Lack of association between electronic health record systems and improvement in use of evidence-based heart failure therapies in outpatient cardiology practices. Clin Cardiol 2012;35(3):187–96. https://doi.org/10.1002/clc.21971.

5. Selvaraj S, Fonarow GC, Sheng S, et al. Association of electronic health record use with quality of care and outcomes in heart failure: an analysis of get with the guidelines- heart failure. J Am Heart Assoc 2018;7(7):1–10. https://doi.org/10.1161/JAHA.117.0081585.

6. Fonarow GC, Albert NM, Curtis AB, et al. Improving evidence-based care for heart failure in outpatient cardiology practices: primary results of the registry to improve the use of evidence-based heart failure therapies in the outpatient setting (IMPROVE HF). Circulation 2010;122(6):585–96. https://doi.org/10.1161/CIRCULATIONAHA.109.934471.

7. Foster M, Albanese C, Chen Q, et al. Heart failure dashboard design and validation to improve care of veterans. Appl Clin Inform 2020;11(1):153–9. https://doi.org/10.1055/s-0040-1701257.

8. Cox ZL, Lewis CM, Lai P, et al. Validation of an automated electronic algorithm and "dashboard" to identify and characterize decompensated heart failure admissions across a medical center. Am Heart J 2017;183:40–8. https://doi.org/10.1016/j.ahj.2016.10.001.

9. Banerjee D, Thompson C, Kell C, et al. An informatics-based approach to reducing heart failure all-cause readmissions: the Stanford heart failure dashboard. J Am Med Inform Assoc 2017;24(3):550–5. https://doi.org/10.1093/jamia/ocw150.

10. SUPPORT-HF2 Investigators and Committees. Home monitoring with IT-supported specialist management versus home monitoring alone in patients with heart failure: design and baseline results of the SUPPORT-HF 2 randomized trial. Am Heart J 2019;208:55–64. https://doi.org/10.1016/j.ahj.2018.09.007.

11. Shameer K, Johnson KW, Yahi A, et al. Predictive modeling of hospital readmission rates using electronic medical record-wide machine learning: a case study using Mount Sinai heart failure cohort. Pac Symp Biocomput 2017;22:276–87.

12. Amarasingham R, Moore BJ, Tabak YP, et al. An automated model to identify heart failure patients at risk for

30-day readmission or death using electronic medical record data. Med Care 2010;48(11):981–8. https://doi.org/10.1097/MLR.0b013e3181ef60d9.

13. Bergquist T, Buie RW, Li K, et al. Heart on FHIR: integrating patient generated data into clinical care to reduce 30 day heart failure readmissions (Extended Abstract). AMIA Ann Symp Proc 2018;2017:2269–73. Available at: http://www.ncbi.nlm.nih.gov/pubmed/29854266%0Ahttp://www.pubmedcentral.nih.gov/articlerender.fcgi?artid=PMC5977686.

14. Jing L, Ulloa Cerna AE, Good CW, et al. A machine learning approach to management of heart failure populations. JACC Hear Fail 2020;8(7):578–87. https://doi.org/10.1016/j.jchf.2020.01.012.

15. Reingold S, Kulstad E. Impact of human factor design on the use of order sets in the treatment of congestive heart failure. Acad Emerg Med 2007;14(11):1097–105. https://doi.org/10.1197/j.aem.2007.05.006.

16. Kitsiou S, Gerber BS, Kansal MM, et al. Patient-centered mobile health technology intervention to improve self-care in patients with chronic heart failure: protocol for a feasibility randomized controlled trial. Contemp Clin Trials 2021;106:106433. https://doi.org/10.1016/j.cct.2021.106433.

17. Ho K, Lauscher HN, Cordeiro J, et al. Testing the feasibility of sensor-based home health monitoring (TEC4Home) to support the convalescence of patients with heart failure: pre–post study. JMIR Form Res 2021;5(6):e24509. https://doi.org/10.2196/24509.

18. Bright TJ, Wong A, Dhurjati R, et al. Effect of clinical decision-support systems. Ann Intern Med 2012; 157(1):29. https://doi.org/10.7326/0003-4819-157-1-201207030-00450.

19. Vader JM, Rue SJ, Louis MS, et al. Clinical decision support for heart failure referral—more work, better outcomes? J Card Fail 2017;23(10):727–8. https://doi.org/10.1016/j.cardfail.2017.08.450.

20. Douthit BJ, Musser RC, Lytle KS, et al. A closer look at the "right" format for clinical decision support: methods for evaluating a storyboard bestpractice advisory. J Pers Med 2020;10(4):1–11. https://doi.org/10.3390/jpm10040142.

21. Blecker S, Austrian JS, Horwitz LI, et al. Interrupting providers with clinical decision support to improve care for heart failure. Int J Med Inform 2019;131:103956. https://doi.org/10.1016/j.ijmedinf.2019.103956.

22. Horsky J, Schiff GD, Johnston D, et al. Interface design principles for useable decision support: a targeted review of best practices for clinical prescribing interventions. J Biomed Inform 2012;45(6):1202–16. https://doi.org/10.1016/j.jbi.2012.09.002.

23. Olakotan OO, Mohd Yusof M. The appropriateness of clinical decision support systems alerts in supporting clinical workflows: a systematic review. Health Inform J 2021;27(2). https://doi.org/10.1177/14604582211007536.

24. Trinkley KE, Blakeslee WW, Matlock DD, et al. Clinician preferences for computerised clinical decision support for medications in primary care: a focus group study. BMJ Health Care Inform 2019;26(1):1–8. https://doi.org/10.1136/bmjhci-2019-000015.

25. Allen LA, Venechuk G, McIlvennan CK, et al. An electronically delivered patient-activation tool for intensification of medications for chronic heart failure with reduced ejection fraction the EPIC-HF trial. Circulation 2021;143:427–37. https://doi.org/10.1161/CIRCULATIONAHA.120.051863.

26. Han HR, Gleason KT, Sun CA, et al. Using patient portals to improve patient outcomes: systematic review. JMIR Hum Factors 2019;6(4):e15038. https://doi.org/10.2196/15038.

27. Stanimirovic D. eHealth Patient Portal - becoming an indispensable public health tool in the time of covid-19. Stud Health Technol Inform 2021;281:880–4. https://doi.org/10.3233/SHTI210305.

28. Ammenwerth E, Neyer S, Hörbst A, et al. Adult patient access to electronic health records. Cochrane Database Syst Rev 2021;2:CD012707. https://doi.org/10.1002/14651858.CD012707.pub2.

29. Reed ME, Huang J, Brand RJ, et al. Patients with complex chronic conditions: health care use and clinical events associated with access to a patient portal. PLoS One 2019;14(6):1–14. https://doi.org/10.1371/journal.pone.0217636.

30. Irizarry T, Shoemake J, Nilsen ML, et al. Patient portals as a tool for health care engagement: a mixed-method study of older adults with varying levels of health literacy and prior patient portal use. J Med Internet Res 2017;19(3):e99. https://doi.org/10.2196/JMIR.7099.

31. Stehlik J, Rodriguez-Correa C, Spertus JA, et al. Implementation of real-time assessment of patient-reported outcomes in a heart failure clinic: a feasibility study. J Card Fail 2017;23(11):813–6. https://doi.org/10.1016/j.cardfail.2017.09.009.

32. Ahmad T, Yamamoto Y, Biswas A, et al. REVeAL-HF: design and rationale of a pragmatic randomized controlled trial embedded within routine clinical practice. JACC Hear Fail 2021;9(6):409–19. https://doi.org/10.1016/j.jchf.2021.03.006.

33. Moore CR, Jain S, Haas S, et al. Ascertaining Framingham heart failure phenotype from inpatient electronic health record data using natural language processing: a multicentre Atherosclerosis Risk in Communities (ARIC) validation study. BMJ Open 2021;11(6):1–7. https://doi.org/10.1136/bmjopen-2020-047356.

34. Kadosh BS, Katz SD, Blecker S. Identification of patients with heart failure in large datasets. Heart Fail Clin 2020;16(4):379–86. https://doi.org/10.1016/j.hfc.2020.05.001.

35. Manrodt C, Curtis AB, Soderlund D, et al. Guideline-concordant-phenotyping: Identifying patient indications for implantable cardioverter defibrillators from

electronic health records. Int J Med Inform 2020; 138:104138. https://doi.org/10.1016/j.ijmedinf.2020. 104138.

36. Thorvaldsen T, Lund LH. Focusing on referral rather than selection for advanced heart failure therapies. Card Fail Rev 2019;5(1):24–6.

37. Lee J, Szeto L, Pasupula DK, et al. Cluster randomized trial examining the impact of automated best practice alert on rates of implantable defibrillator therapy. Circ Cardiovasc Qual Outcomes 2019;12(6):1–9. https://doi.org/10.1161/CIRCOUTCOMES.118.005024.

38. Howlett J, Morrin L, Fortin M, et al. End-of-life planning in heart failure: it should be the end of the beginning. Can J Cardiol 2010;26(3):135–41. https://doi.org/10.1016/S0828-282X(10)70351-2.

39. Kalra A, Bhatt DL, Wei J, et al. Electronic health records and outpatient cardiovascular disease care delivery: insights from the American College of Cardiology's PINNACLE India Quality Improvement Program (PIQIP). Indian Heart J 2018;70(5):750–2. https://doi.org/10.1016/j.ihj.2018.03.002.

40. Tu SW, Martins S, Oshiro C, et al. Automating performance measures and clinical practice guidelines: differences and complementarities. AMIA Annu Symp Proc 2016;2016:1199–208. Available at: http://www.ncbi.nlm.nih.gov/pubmed/28269917. January 29, 2018.

41. Riggio JM, Sorokin R, Moxey ED, et al. Effectiveness of a clinical-decision-support system in improving compliance with cardiac-care quality measures and supporting resident training. Acad Med 2009;84(12):1719–26. https://doi.org/10.1097/ACM.0b013e3181bf51d6.

42. Guidi G, Pettenati MC, Melillo P, et al. A machine learning system to improve heart failure patient assistance. IEEE J Biomed Health Inf 2014;18(6):1750–6. https://doi.org/10.1109/JBHI.2014.2337752.

43. Gorlicki J, Boubaya M, Cottin Y, et al. Patient care pathways in acute heart failure and their impact on in-hospital mortality, a French national prospective survey. IJC Hear Vasc 2020;26:100448. https://doi.org/10.1016/j.ijcha.2019.100448.

44. Kul S, Barbieri A, Milan E, et al. Effects of care pathways on the in-hospital treatment of heart failure: a systematic review. BMC Cardiovasc Disord 2012; 12. https://doi.org/10.1186/1471-2261-12-81.

45. Van Stipdonk AMW, Schretlen S, Dohmen W, et al. Development and implementation of a cardiac resynchronisation therapy care pathway: Improved process and reduced resource use. BMJ Open Qual 2021;10(1):1–8. https://doi.org/10.1136/bmjoq-2020-001072.

46. Ranjan A, Tarigopula L, Srivastava RK, et al. Effectiveness of the clinical pathway in the management of congestive heart failure. South Med J 2003;96(7): 661–3. https://doi.org/10.1097/01.SMJ.0000060581. 77206.ED.

47. Dhaliwal JS, Goss F, Whittington MD, et al. Reduced admission rates and resource utilization for chest pain patients using an electronic health record-embedded clinical pathway in the emergency department. J Am Coll Emerg Physicians Open 2020;1(6):1602–13. https://doi.org/10.1002/emp2.12308.

48. Patel H, Virapongse A, Baduashvili A, et al. Implementing a COVID-19 discharge pathway to improve patient safety. Am J Med Qual 2021;36(2):84–9. https://doi.org/10.1097/01.JMQ.0000735436.50361.79.

49. Amarasingham R, Patel PC, Toto K, et al. Allocating scarce resources in real-time to reduce heart failure readmissions: a prospective, controlled study. BMJ Qual Saf 2013;22(12):998–1005. https://doi.org/10.1136/bmjqs-2013-001901.

50. Fonarow GC, Yancy CW, Albert NM, et al. Improving the use of evidence-based heart failure therapies in the outpatient setting: the IMPROVE HF performance improvement registry. Am Heart J 2007;154(1):12–38. https://doi.org/10.1016/j.ahj.2007.03.030.

51. Walsh MN, Yancy CW, Albert NM, et al. Electronic health records and quality of care for heart failure. Am Heart J 2010;159(4):635–42.e1. https://doi.org/10.1016/j.ahj.2010.01.006.

52. Evans RS, Kfoury AG, Horne BD, et al. Clinical decision support to efficiently identify patients eligible for advanced heart failure therapies. J Card Fail 2017; 23(10):719–26. https://doi.org/10.1016/j.cardfail.2017. 08.449.

53. Bhakta P, Biswas BK, Banerjee B. Peripartum cardiomyopathy: review of the literature. Yonsei Med J 2007; 48(5):731–47. https://doi.org/10.3349/ymj.2007.48.5. 731.

54. Miller RJH, Bell A, Aggarwal S, et al. Computerized electronic order set: use and outcomes for heart failure following hospitalization. CJC Open 2020;2(6): 497–505. https://doi.org/10.1016/j.cjco.2020.06.009.

55. Krive J, Shoolin JS, Zink SD. Effectiveness of evidence-based congestive heart failure (CHF) CPOE order sets measured by health outcomes. AMIA Annu Symp Proc 2014;2014:815–24. Available at: http://www.ncbi.nlm.nih.gov/pubmed/25954388. January 30, 2018.

56. Ballard DJ, Ogola G, Fleming NS, et al. Impact of a standardized heart failure order set on mortality, readmission, and quality and costs of care. Int J Qual Health Care 2010;22(6):437–44. https://doi.org/10. 1093/intqhc/mzq051.

57. Small RS, Wickemeyer W, Germany R, et al. Changes in intrathoracic impedance are associated with subsequent risk of hospitalizations for acute decompensated heart failure: clinical utility of implanted device monitoring without a patient alert. J Card Fail 2009;15(6):475–81. https://doi.org/10. 1016/j.cardfail.2009.01.012.

58. Whellan DJ, Ousdigian KT, Al-Khatib SM, et al. Combined heart failure device diagnostics identify

patients at higher risk of subsequent heart failure hospitalizations. results from PARTNERS HF (Program to access and review trending information and evaluate correlation to symptoms in patients with heart failure) study. J Am Coll Cardiol 2010; 55(17):1803–10. https://doi.org/10.1016/j.jacc.2009. 11.089.

59. Abraham WT, Adamson PB, Bourge RC, et al. Wireless pulmonary artery haemodynamic monitoring in chronic heart failure: a randomised controlled trial. Lancet 2011;377(9766):658–66. https://doi.org/10. 1016/S0140-6736(11)60101-3.

60. Park C, Otobo E, Ullman J, et al. Impact on readmission reduction among heart failure patients using digital health monitoring: feasibility and adoptability study. JMIR Med Inform 2019;7(4):1–10. https://doi. org/10.2196/13353.

61. Kallmerten PS, Chia LR, Jakub K, et al. Patient portal use by adults with heart failure. Comput Inform Nurs 2021;39(8):418–31. https://doi.org/10.1097/ cin.0000000000000733.

62. Earnest MA, Ross SE, Wittevrongel L, et al. Use of a patient-accessible electronic medical record in a practice for congestive heart failure: patient and physician experiences. J Am Med Inform Assoc 2004;11(5): 410–7. https://doi.org/10.1197/jamia.M1479.

63. Dang S, Siddharthan K, Ruiz DI, et al. Evaluating an electronic health record intervention for management of heart failure among veterans. Telemed J E

Health 2018;24(12):1006–13. https://doi.org/10. 1089/tmj.2017.0307.

64. Freise L, Neves AL, Flott K, et al. Assessment of patients' ability to review electronic health record information to identify potential errors: cross-sectional web-based survey. JMIR Form Res 2021;5(2):1–10. https://doi.org/10.2196/19074.

65. Mondesir FL, Zickmund SL, Yang S, et al. Patient perspectives on the completion and use of patient-reported outcome surveys in routine clinical care for heart failure. Circ Cardiovasc Qual Outcomes 2020;13(9):695–7. https://doi.org/10.1161/ CIRCOUTCOMES.120.007027.

66. Atasoy H, Greenwood BN, McCullough JS. The digitization of patient care: a review of the effects of electronic health records on health care quality and utilization. Annu Rev Public Health 2019;40:487–500. https://doi.org/10.1146/annurev-publhealth-040218-044206.

67. Silva Almodóvar A, Nahata MC. Implementing clinical decision support tools and pharmacovigilance to reduce the use of potentially harmful medications and health care costs in adults with heart failure. Front Pharmacol 2021;12:1–7. https://doi.org/10. 3389/fphar.2021.612941.

68. Levick DL, Stern G, Meyerhoefer CD, et al. Reducing unnecessary testing in a CPOE system through implementation of a targeted CDS intervention. BMC Med Inform Decis Mak 2013;13(1):1–7. https://doi.org/10.1186/1472-6947-13-43.

Telehealth in Heart Failure

Savitri Fedson, MD, MA[a,b,c], Biykem Bozkurt, MD, PhD[a,c,d],*

KEYWORDS

- Telehealth • Heart failure • Telemedicine • Remote monitoring

KEY POINTS

- Telehealth is critically important in heart failure, and represents an opportunity to enhance timely access and follow-up, utilization of technology for diagnostic and management strategies, individualize management, increase opportunities for multidisciplinary care, eliminate social and medical barriers to care, and implement complementary management strategies.
- Telemedical interventional management strategies and telemonitoring have been associated with a reduction in heart failure-related hospitalizations and heart failure-related mortality.
- Despite all the potential benefits of expanded access, telehealth may have limitations especially for vulnerable populations, who are at risk for less access to health care, such as the elderly, those experiencing homelessness or housing instability, migrant workers, may have limitations and barriers in their access to virtual health. Every effort should be conducted for equal access to telehealth, digital technologies, and virtual platform for health equity.

INTRODUCTION

Telehealth is the delivery of health care services and health care information whereby patients and providers are separated by a physical distance. This ranges from the use of technology to send patient data back to providers, to the use of virtual clinic visits with video streaming. The use of some forms of telehealth in cardiology is longstanding. Holter monitors have been in use since 1949, implantable loop recorders since the early 1990s, and the ability to remotely monitor implantable cardioverter-defibrillators is likewise well established. Beyond this, telemedicine has been routinely used by emergency medical services, transmitting electrocardiograms (ECG) to local emergency departments from the field for triage and earlier activation of cardiac catheterization laboratories for acute ST-elevation myocardial infarctions. Despite this, in 2019 only 8% of the U.S. population regularly used telehealth for their formal health care services,[1] while at the same time telehealth technologies with mobile health applications and fitness trackers (m-Health) are were used by up to 60% of the population.[2] The COVID-19 pandemic catapulted telemedicine into the mainstream with the necessary transition to a telehealth-based health care delivery model. While this has shown the potential for the delivery of quality care,[3] it has also underscored some of the ongoing challenges to provide health care with mixed modalities.

The need to more widely incorporate telehealth into the management of patients with heart failure (HF) may represent an opportunity to integrate conventional face-to-face provider–patient encounters with complementary management strategies.[4] HF is a chronic progressive disorder that affects nearly 6 million in the United States alone, and 30 million worldwide. With increasing prevalence in the elderly and aging populations, HF management faces challenges that arise from the constellation of symptoms of intravascular volume and congestion, frailty, and cognitive impairment that accompany this disease. Hospital admissions contribute to nearly 80% of the cost burden of HF in the United States and are additionally associated with increased mortality and morbidity. HF has qualities that would be well suited to a

[a] Michael E DeBakey VA Medical Center, Houston, TX, USA; [b] Center for Medical Ethics and Health Policy, Baylor College of Medicine, One Baylor Plaza, Houston, TX 77030, USA; [c] Winters Center for Heart Failure Research, One Baylor Plaza, Houston, TX 77030, USA; [d] Cardiovascular Research Institute, Baylor College of Medicine, One Baylor Plaza, Houston, TX 77030, USA
* Corresponding author. MEDVAMC, 2002 Holcombe Boulevard, Houston, TX 77030.
E-mail address: bbozkurt@bcm.edu

Heart Failure Clin 18 (2022) 213–221
https://doi.org/10.1016/j.hfc.2021.12.001
1551-7136/22/Published by Elsevier Inc.

heartfailure.theclinics.com

telehealth-based approach to health care. It is an episodic disease, with periods of stability punctuated by decompensation and increasing symptoms requiring either medication adjustment, or hospitalization. Each subsequent hospitalization then is accompanied by increased risk for recurrent decompensation and increased mortality, in part because of the transition of care at this pivotal time, and the need for the reinstitution of medication, or medication titration. Relying on face-to-face encounters for this is often impractical, yet there is a need for clinician–patient interaction to achieve this. Furthermore, telehealth can help with access for follow-up for patients who do not have easy access to a health care facility due to distance, transportation limitations, other social or health reasons, unavailability of a specialist and or clinician as long as infrastructure can be supported in an equitable manner.

Despite overwhelming data supporting guideline-directed medical therapy (GDMT) for HF with reduced ejection fraction, the ability to achieve target doses of medication, much less simultaneous use of these classes of medicine has been difficult.[5] Disease management programs have using face-to-face strategies are time and labor-intensive and are often challenging likewise for patients who have limitations with ambulation, transportation, or geographic proximity to their provider. In some studies, slightly over half of those patients readmitted to a hospital within 30 days of hospital discharge had not seen a health care provider since their discharge.[6]

Different strategies to supplement the traditional provider–patient encounter have been studied, with a broad range of outcomes, but with varied benefits in terms of hospitalization or mortality. Some of the challenges of interpreting the studies of telehealth interventions are the varied approaches, which have been used, differences in the study population and the different health care systems they are embedded within. Some interventions have used structured telephone support (STS) which typically uses question prompts for patients about symptoms and health statistics, prompting alerts to providers according to their response. Others use telemonitoring (TM) relying on the transmission of physiologic data to the provider. There has been a trend toward decreasing HF-related hospitalizations and HF-related mortality in many of these trials, with greater benefit demonstrated when there was the incorporation of greater than 3 physiologic data sent via TM.[7–12] The telehealth interventions have demonstrated improvements in HF-related quality of life (QoL) measures, and reduction in depressive symptoms. What comprises these interventions need to be examined more closely.

Forms of Telehealth Commonly used in Heart Failure

Telehealth is critically important in HF, and represents an opportunity to enhance timely access and follow-up, utilization of technology for diagnostic and management strategies, individualize management, increase opportunities for multidisciplinary care, eliminate social and medical barriers to care, and implement complementary management strategies.

Telehealth can be largely divided into 3 areas: clinician-to-clinician communication; the patient interacting with mobile health technologies (m-Health), and lastly clinician–patient interaction (**Fig. 1**; **Table 1**).

Clinician-to-Clinician

The role of telehealth in clinician–clinician communication, or teleconsultation has advanced with technologies, moving beyond standard telephones to e-mail communication, video conferencing, and sharing of video data. These consultations can provide access to HF specialists who can remotely view diagnostic data, whether from standard echocardiogram platforms, or the images from hand-held scanners. They can also form the basis of "hub and spoke" models of care as has been modeled both with HF and with the management of patients with ventricular assist devices (VADs). Integrating teleconsultation forms of telehealth in HF can assist with management during the most vulnerable period of transition from the hospital back to the community-based providers. The varied modalities that comprise telehealth can be incorporated into a model of HF management that then makes use of the concept of the Heart Team, coordinating the efforts of all the clinicians involved in the care of these patients during these transitions of care. E-health, through the sharing of medical records, can incorporate triggered reminders or alerts for the up-titration or initiation of GDMT, to follow-up with laboratory testing or parenteral iron administration. Not only might this work for communication with HF specialists but also for other members of the management team such as pharmacists and palliative care specialists.[13] The efficacy of this type of intervention is currently being studied in the Spanish Heart failure Events reduction with Remote Monitoring and eHealth Support (HERMeS) trial.

There is a supply mismatch between the number of advanced HF cardiologists and the number of patients with HF of all stages. Telehealth

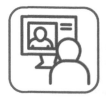

Clinician-to-clinician communication

- Specialty consultation
- Multidisciplinary group consultation
- Care Coordination
- Electronic-consults
- Stored data interpretation

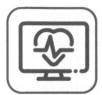

Patient interaction with health technologies

- Remote monitoring (invasive and non-invasive)
- Wearable devices
- Smart-phone technology
- Digital technology

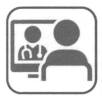

Clinician-to-patient interaction

- Virtual visits (e.g. outpatient visits, post-discharge follow-up)
- Secure messaging
- Interpretation of health information virtually (e.g. test results, mobile health applications , remote monitoring)
- Multi-disciplinary clinician-to-patient interaction (e.g. transplant teams, cardiac rehabilitation, palliative care, social work)

Fig. 1. Forms of telehealth commonly used in heart failure.

e-consultation can allow those in different communities to have access to providers who can suggest medical optimization, or importantly when it might be appropriate to refer to an advanced HF center.

Patient-Data Capture and Remote Monitoring Through Health Technologies

Remote monitoring (RM) allows for the transfer of patient-generated data from the patient to the health care team in a timely manner, across distances. Currently, the most widespread example of this is through the monitoring of ICD/CRT-D for arrhythmias. The monitoring of thoracic impedance is also available in some devices, but not as integrated into the care team algorithms.

Implantable pulmonary artery sensors (Cardio-MEMS), in particular, have been shown to decrease HF-related hospitalizations at 6 months, in patients with NYHA III irrespective of ejection fraction in the CHAMPION trial. In addition, there was a benefit in QoL as evidenced by decreased MLWHFQ scores at 6 and 12 months.[14,15] The CHAMPION trial was nonblinded, however, and there was a different level of patient contact between the 2 arms, reinforcing the importance of the human element of processing and responding to the patient-derived data. In the recently published GUIDE-HF trial, implantation of pulmonary artery pressure monitor, in patients with NYHA functional class II–IV HF, with either a recent HF hospitalization or elevated natriuretic peptides did not result in a lower composite endpoint rate of mortality and total HF events compared with the control group in the overall study analysis.[16] However, a pre–COVID-19 impact analysis indicated a possible benefit of hemodynamic-guided management on the primary outcome in the pre–COVID-19 period, primarily driven by a lower HF hospitalization rate compared with the control group.[16]

The assessment of lung congestion using thoracic impedance measures, either with the wearable remote dielectric sensing (ReDS) or the implanted impedance monitors linked to cardiac implantable electric devices, has not been shown to lead to significant decreases in HF hospitalization although more recent studies are more promising, and are ongoing. Part of the limitation of benefit may be linked to the role of patient action to put on the device or to deliberately transmit data.

Wearable devices also permit RM. These are noninvasive sensors that collect data and store them for clinical decision making later. Some are prescribed devices, such as Holter monitors, ambulatory blood pressure monitors, while others are products advertised directly to consumers trying to track or improve their health. m-Health, using smartphone applications also has significant potential uses in HF, with applications tailored to help with medication adherence through automated reminders, monitoring of daily activity.[2,17] However, the integrity of publicly available

Table 1 Forms of telehealth	
Types of Telehealth	**Explanation**
Telehealth	Provision of health care remotely by means of telecommunications technology
Telemedicine	Use of telecommunications to deliver health care at a distance (implies clinical services)
m-Health	Mobile computing, wireless communication, sensors, mobile health apps, social media; electronic stethoscope, hand-held ultrasound
e-Health	Information and communication technology in support of health and health care-related fields, shared electronic medical record
Digital Health	E-learning, remote monitoring, telephonic interventions
Remote Monitoring	Weights, BP, ICD, implantable PA pressure monitoring, thoracic impedance
Teleconsultation	Communication between clinicians across distances, using telehealth

physiologic tools is not without error, especially at higher heart rates, and in those with darker skin for pulse oximetry.[18] Moreover, there is little regulatory oversight for these m-Health applications. The U.S. Food and Drug Administration does regulate medical devices, but states that the intention of the m-Health app will determine whether it qualifies as a device to be regulated, and the potential risk to patients. Examples of m-Health that might be regulated include electronic stethoscopes or those that monitor heart rate variability from an electrocardiograph.[2,19]

Clinician-to-Patient Communication

Clinician–patient communication using telehealth has historically been based on telephone support,

either informally organized or structured (STS) as in the trials. This can involve the incorporation of additional input from RM, or laboratory data, but is both time and personnel intensive. One of the comments regarding the impracticability of the TIM-HF2[9] study was the presence of 24-h coverage of the communication lines to patients. With the social distancing practices during the COVID-19 pandemic, health care delivery relied on telehealth structures between providers and patients with the addition of the virtual video clinic (VVC) visit. The VVC can be based solely on information gathered at the time of the encounter, or can also include additional RM or laboratory data.

The VVC has been the focus of discussion about telehealth, but it is only one piece of health care delivery. There are tips for the preparation of the visit, for the patient as well as for the provider to improve the quality of these visits.[20,21] These also include suggestions on how to create rapport over distance, how to conduct a limited physical examination, and the chance to include advance care planning topics (**Tables 2–4**). The possibility of incorporating the family or caregivers in the clinic appointments can add an important source of information about medical compliance, under-reporting of symptoms and functional status, and when nonmedical factors might need to be addressed. Institutions, such as the Veteran's Health Administration (VHA) and Kaiser Permanente were adopters of this virtual platform before the pandemic and provided guidance for structure. The clinical preparation before VVC is no less than for in-person visits as this might require review of m-Health data from other platforms, and often requires the online real-time assessment of vitals by the patient themselves. In a recent randomized controlled trial, outpatient telecare with nurse-led noninvasive assessments reduced the risk of HF hospitalization rates during 12-month follow-up among patients with HF and left ventricular ejection fraction ≤49% and history of acute HF within the last 6 months when compared with usual care.[22] According to the study protocol, the nurse-led telehealth intervention included the assessment of presence and intensity of HF symptoms according to NYHA class using predefined questionnaires, measurements of impedance cardiography or thoracic impedance, and treatment recommendations formulated by a cardiologist.[22]

m-Health can also be effective in providing education to patients about symptoms, possible exacerbating factors, and self-management strategies. These can include educational media, text message reminders, or links to other social media sources. Furthermore, m-Health can be used to

Table 2 Physical examination	
Vital Signs	Weight, Blood Pressure, Temperature, Oxygen Saturation
Skin assessment	New Bruising, rashes
Head, Eyes, Ears, Nose, Throat	Assess symmetry of eye movements, hearing, appearance of scleral icterus
Cardiovascular	
Neck	Jugular Venous distension Bendopnea
	Lower extremity edema, ulcers
Fitness	Sit to stand, gait assessment
Limitations	Touch sensation of skin temperature, perfusion

Table 3 Communication tools for virtual visit	
Communication Concepts	Example
Naming	"It sounds like your symptoms are worse."
Understanding	"This helps me understand what you just told me."
Respecting	"I can see that you have really made efforts to improve your diet."
Supporting	"I will work with you to try to get you what you need."
Exploring	"Could you tell me a little more about what you mean when you said that...?"

support decision aids for advanced HF options and for advance care planning, permitting patients and families time to explore their preferences before a provider–patient interaction. These interventions have been studied, again without robust findings but demonstrate the feasibility of integrating these into clinical management.[23]

Telehealth-Cardiac Rehabilitation

Cardio-pulmonary rehabilitation can be provided through telehealth and video visits. Home-based cardiac rehabilitation has been suggested as an alternative for traditional center-based cardiac rehabilitation to help increase access, participation and adherence[24–26] Programs have successfully used components of telehealth to further improve on these home-based programs. Video conferencing can permit the exercise physiologist to provide immediate feedback and demonstration for exercise techniques; assessment of frailty and instability can be assessed watching patients rise from chairs or walk in front of the camera.[27]

Challenges to Telehealth Implementation

For all the potential benefits of expanded access, there remain limitations of telehealth. Those vulnerable populations, who are at risk for less access to health care, such as the elderly, those experiencing homelessness or housing instability, migrant workers, are also vulnerable in their access to virtual health. They may have limited proficiency with technology, or limited broadband access, or few minutes for a telephone-only plan.[28] For patients with dementia or impaired hearing, communication often relies on nonverbal cues such as lip reading, body and facial expressions, which are limited over video interfaces. The delay or lag in the electrical interface, interruptions, or ambient noises can also worsen this communication and lead to misunderstandings, frustrations, or an unwillingness to rely on these methods of care delivery. Every effort should be conducted for equal access to telehealth, digital technologies, and virtual platform for health equity. Health care systems should invest in technologies and provide equipment and connectivity to ensure that telehealth does not widen health disparities.

Limitations of Telehealth

For telehealth to be successful, patients and clinicians must be willing and able, and the technology must be available and effective. Some patients and clinicians, especially those with limited infrastructure or access to technology and or virtual connectivity, limited technology comfort may be reluctant to use telehealth. Some patients and clinicians may have physical barriers to use telehealth due to hearing, visual, or other differences. Some may be reluctant to use telehealth due to privacy concerns. Importantly utilization of virtual interactions in lieu of face-to-face

Table 4
Pros: Cons virtual visit

	Pros	Cons
Access	Improved for those with limited mobility, distance, transportation, child-care needs	Requires technologic literacy, broadband, potential lack of privacy
Environment	Can alert providers to potential safety issues in environment; can "see" the medicine bottles	Lack of privacy; unwillingness to reveal one's home environment
Care Transitions	Continuity of care more easily	
Physical Examination/Distance	Observation of breathing, orthopnea/bendopnea, visual inspection of neck veins, leg edema, incorporation of physiologic data from remote monitoring	Lack of "therapeutic" touch; Challenging for people relying on nonverbal cues; limited ability to complete examination (skin temperature, pulse characteristics)

visits create concerns regarding lack of ability to perform a full physical examination, have an opportunity for more in-person interaction. Geographic and financial challenges to access Wi-Fi connectivity, computer, smartphone, network, or software platforms remain as major limitations for vulnerable populations creating health inequity. Furthermore, virtual visits do not allow immediate intervention with intravenous therapies, further diagnostic imaging or laboratory studies, or admission to a hospital for higher level of care that may be commonly used in patients with HF. This is a significant concern for patients with worsening symptoms and or hemodynamic instability when an in-person visit may be better than a virtual visit. Due to the limitations of virtual visits, there are also concerns regarding missing important findings that may not be easily visible or discernible by virtual visits, such as subtle changes in physical examination findings, vital signs, or laboratory markers. Actively worsening patients who may require higher levels of care such as additional laboratory and diagnostic tests, intravenous or interventional treatment, and or admission to the hospital may require in-person visits rather than telehealth. Patients with advanced HF symptoms may need to be considered for hybrid models of telehealth including postdischarge telehealth visits, combined with in-person visits when symptoms are worse and or when higher level of care is needed.

Privacy

Additionally, telehealth, and indeed, electronic communication has permeated society, but it is important not to forget the risk to patient privacy, especially on unsecured platforms or networks. The concern for privacy is not only for the patient but also for the provider, because there is no certainty as to whom might be in the virtual clinic room, especially if there is no video feed. There are preferred platforms to use for telehealth encounters, some designed solely for this use, requiring password protection.

The coordinated use of different modalities of telehealth, using the electronic health record to identify at-risk patients, RM for biometric data, and telephone follow-up to maximize medicine titration can be conducted, even before the COVID-19 pandemic.[29] However, as was noted in this single-center study, the patients who participated were younger.

Jurisdiction

One of the additional challenges to telemedicine is the jurisdiction of medical licensure and provider reimbursement. Where does the provider–patient relationship start? In general, for there to be a provider–patient relationship (PPR), a person must "present" themselves for treatment or advice, the provider then provides advice, which the person, now a patient, relies, and acts on. These comprise the relationship but historically, this starts with a traditional face-to-face encounter. It was only with the COVID-19 pandemic that there was an easing of this restriction to allow the initiation of PPR relations to be via telemedicine and temporary waivers in some regulation of telehealth services. Specifically, the need for providers to hold licenses in the states in which they are telepracticing have been waived, whereas before this, to provide telehealth services, a provider had to be licensed in that state, or be in one of the states that grant reciprocity, or practicing though the Veterans Health Administration (VHA) which allows for clinician license portability. Even before COVID-19, there was an increased expansion for the reimbursement of telehealth encounters, specifically for end-stage renal disease, stroke, and substance abuse.[30] As the increased update of VVC visits and other telehealth options, some states have made legislative changes that make permanent some of the pandemic waivers.

RM is not considered to be telehealth; however, to then act or provide advice based on these data is a form of telehealth and would be governed by license restrictions; this has created limitations for provider accessibility in the past. One potential drawback of the patient-derived data using m-Health apps is how to best coordinate provider responses. What is the responsibility of a provider to react to, or act on data that may be inaccurate? Will delays in provider response lead to psychological stress? These are yet unanswered questions and ones that will be challenging given the constraints of both time and personnel that already exist within HF management teams.

Additional barriers to the implantation of telehealth in HF will be provider reimbursement. At present, simple telephone visits, which may be as lengthy as VVC, do not have the same reimbursement, which might push providers aware of those patients who prefer the more simple technology of a telephone.

Because of the clinical challenges of frequent medication titration in the HF population, the social determinants of health can have significant repercussions for models of telehealth, and as telehealth continues to expand there will have to be targeted approaches to help overcome some of the barriers to implementation, which have the potential to worsen some of these disparities. For example, those experiencing homelessness or unstable living conditions might not have access to reliable networks or personal technology to implement the full use of monitoring m-Health applications or e-health education platforms for triggered reminders for medications adherence, or responses to biometric data. Data from experience with telehealth during the COVID-19 pandemic suggest that patients who are older, single, African-American, or of lower socioeconomic status by education and income were less likely to use VVC than telephone visits.[25]

If the HeartTeam relies heavily on these technologies, then a cohort of patients risks falling further behind. As noted earlier, HF is associated with cognitive dysfunction, which can also limit the patient-technology interaction or feeling of ease.[31] The challenge of an appropriate digital prescription is a new element for the HF provider.

Future of telehealth will include the increased use of artificial intelligence in pattern recognition and interpretation of data. Managing the volumes of patient-derived data and either creating alerts for patients directly or to providers is already in practice for implantable PA pressure and thoracic impedance monitors. As more platforms transmit data, integration of these data sets into patient-specific predictions will be a goal. Artificial intelligence may also be used to discover newer tools to help predict compensation in the telehealth area. An example of this might be the analysis of voice characteristics over the telephone to predict decompensation and hospitalization.[32]

Diabetes mellitus is an example of a disease that has been transformed using m-Health with at-home glucose monitoring. HF management has relied on the bathroom scale for years, combined with patient education to also allow for sliding scale diuretic adjustments, but weight changes may seem too late in the spiral of decompensation to prevent hospitalizations effectively. The self-administration of subcutaneous furosemide might be an option for select patients after the integration of their physiologic data. Home-based services, such as phlebotomy for laboratory testing, using home health aides, or nurses as physician extenders, who might be able to assist vulnerable patients with health care visits, being the eyes, ears and literal hands of the HF provider might be a mechanism to combine technology with patient care.

SUMMARY

In HF care, telehealth represents a very important opportunity to enhance timely access and follow-up, expand the utilization of technology platforms for diagnostic and management strategies, individualize management, increase opportunities for multidisciplinary care coordination, and help implement complementary management strategies.

CLINICS CARE POINTS

- Clinicians and health networks should examine strategies to incorporate telehealth in the management of patients with HF. Telehealth represents an opportunity to enhance timely access and follow-up, utilization of technology for diagnostic and management strategies, individualize management, increase opportunities for multidisciplinary care, and implement complementary management strategies.

- Telemedical interventional management strategies and TM have been associated with a reduction in HF-related hospitalizations and HF-related mortality.
- Health care systems should invest in technologies and providing equipment and connectivity to ensure that telehealth does not widen health disparities. Despite all the potential benefits of expanded access, telehealth may have limitations especially for vulnerable populations, who are at risk for less access to health care.
- Patients with advanced HF symptoms may need to be considered for hybrid models of telehealth including postdischarge telehealth visits, combined with in-person visits when symptoms are worse and or when higher level of care is needed.

DISCLOSURE

B. Bozkurt: Consultation for Bayer, Astra Zeneca, Vifor, Relypsa and scPharmaceuticals, Clinical Events Committee for Guide-HF Trial Abbott Pharmaceuticals, Data Safety Monitoring Board for Anthem Trial by LivaNova Pharmaceuticals. S. Fedson: has nothing to disclose.

REFERENCES

1. Vogels EA. About one-in-five Americans use a smart watch or fitness tracker. Pew Research Center. 9-19-2021. Available at: https://www.pewresearch.org/fact-tank/2020/01/09/about-one-in-five-americans-use-a-smart-watch-or-fitness-tracker/. Accessed December 28, 2021.
2. MacKinnon GE, Brittain EL. Mobile Health Technologies in Cardiopulmonary Disease. Chest 2020; 157(3):654–64.
3. Analysis of UDS Clinical Quality Measure Performance by Health Center Telehealth Use by Health Information Technology and Evaluation Center. September 22 2020. Available at: https://hiteqcenter.org/Resources/Telehealth-Telemedicine/analysis-of-uds-clinical-quality-measure-performance-by-health-center-telehealth-use. Accessed December 28, 2021.
4. Seferovic PM, Ponikowski P, Anker SD, et al. Clinical practice update on heart failure 2019: pharmacotherapy, procedures, devices and patient management. An expert consensus meeting report of the Heart Failure Association of the European Society of Cardiology. Eur J Heart Fail 2019;21(10):1169–86.
5. Thibodeau JT, Gorodeski EZ. Telehealth for uptitration of guideline-directed medical therapy in heart failure. Circulation 2020;142(16):1507–9.
6. Black JT, Romano PS, Sadeghi B, et al. A remote monitoring and telephone nurse coaching intervention to reduce readmissions among patients with heart failure: study protocol for the better effectiveness after transition - heart failure (BEAT-HF) randomized controlled trial. Trials 2014;15:124.
7. Yun JE, Park JE, Park HY, et al. Comparative effectiveness of telemonitoring versus usual care for heart failure: a systematic review and meta-analysis. J Card Fail 2018;24(1):19–28.
8. Galinier M, Roubille F, Berdague P, et al. Telemonitoring versus standard care in heart failure: a randomised multicentre trial. Eur J Heart Fail 2020;22(6):985–94.
9. Koehler F, Koehler K, Deckwart O, et al. Efficacy of telemedical interventional management in patients with heart failure (TIM-HF2): a randomised, controlled, parallel-group, unmasked trial. Lancet 2018;392(10152):1047–57.
10. Inglis SC, Clark RA, Cleland JG. Telemonitoring in patients with heart failure. N Engl J Med 2011; 364(11):1078–9.
11. Ong MK, Romano PS, Edgington S, et al. Effectiveness of remote patient monitoring after discharge of hospitalized patients with heart failure: the better effectiveness after transition – heart failure (BEAT-HF) randomized clinical trial. JAMA Intern Med 2016;176(3):310–8.
12. Inglis SC, Clark RA, Dierckx R, et al. Structured telephone support or non-invasive telemonitoring for patients with heart failure. Cochrane Database Syst Rev 2015;10:CD007228.
13. Huitema AA, Harkness K, Heckman GA, et al. The spoke-hub-and-node model of integrated heart failure care. Can J Cardiol 2018;34(7):863–70.
14. Abraham WT, Stevenson LW, Bourge RC, et al. Sustained efficacy of pulmonary artery pressure to guide adjustment of chronic heart failure therapy: complete follow-up results from the CHAMPION randomised trial. Lancet 2016;387(10017):453–61.
15. Adamson PB, Abraham WT, Stevenson LW, et al. Pulmonary artery pressure-guided heart failure management reduces 30-day readmissions. Circ Heart Fail 2016;9(6).
16. Lindenfeld J, Zile MR, Desai AS, et al. Haemodynamic-guided management of heart failure (GUIDE-HF): a randomised controlled trial. Lancet 2021;398(10304):991–1001.
17. Singhal A, Cowie MR. The role of wearables in heart failure. Curr Heart Fail Rep 2020;17(4):125–32.
18. Nguyen HH, Silva JN. Use of smartphone technology in cardiology. Trends Cardiovasc Med 2016; 26(4):376–86.

19. FDA. Policy for device software functions and mobile medical applications. 9-10-2021. Available at: https://www.fda.gov/regulatory-information/search-fda-guidance-documents/policy-device-software-functions-and-mobile-medical-applications. Accessed December 28, 2021.

20. Gorodeski EZ, Goyal P, Cox ZL, et al. Virtual visits for care of patients with heart failure in the Era of COVID-19: A Statement from the Heart Failure Society of America. J Card Fail 2020;26(6):448–56.

21. Orso F, Migliorini M, Herbst A, et al. Protocol for telehealth evaluation and follow-up of patients with chronic heart failure during the COVID-19 Pandemic. J Am Med Dir Assoc 2020;21(12): 1803–7.

22. Krzesiński P, Jankowska EA, Siebert J, et al. Effects of an outpatient intervention comprising nurse-led non-invasive assessments, telemedicine support and remote cardiologists' decisions in patients with heart failure (AMULET study): a randomised controlled trial. Eur J Heart Fail 2021. https://doi.org/10.1002/ejhf.2358. Epub ahead of print. PMID: 34617373.

23. Allida S, Du H, Xu X, et al. mHealth education interventions in heart failure. Cochrane Database Syst Rev 2020;7:CD011845.

24. Thomas RJ, Beatty AL, Beckie TM, et al. Home-based cardiac rehabilitation: a scientific statement from the American Association of Cardiovascular and Pulmonary Rehabilitation, the American Heart Association, and the American College of Cardiology. J Am Coll Cardiol 2019;74(1):133–53.

25. Sammour Y, Spertus JA, Shatla I, et al. Comparison of video and telephone visits in outpatients with heart failure. Am J Cardiol 2021;158:153–6.

26. Bozkurt B, Fonarow GC, Goldberg LR, et al. Cardiac rehabilitation for patients with heart failure: JACC Expert Panel. J Am Coll Cardiol 2021;77(11): 1454–69.

27. Bryant MS, Fedson SE, Sharafkhaneh A. Using Telehealth Cardiopulmonary Rehabilitation during the COVID-19 Pandemic. J Med Syst 2020;44(7):125.

28. Lam K, Lu AD, Shi Y, et al. Assessing telemedicine unreadiness among older adults in the United States During the COVID-19 Pandemic. JAMA Intern Med 2020;180(10):1389–91.

29. Desai AS, Maclean T, Blood AJ, et al. Remote optimization of guideline-directed medical therapy in patients with heart failure with reduced ejection fraction. JAMA Cardiol 2020;5(12):1430–4.

30. Latifi R, Doarn CR, Merrell RC, eds. Telemedicine, Telehealth and Telepresence: Principles, Strategies, Applications, and New Directions 1st ed. 2021.

31. Rodriguez JA, Betancourt JR, Sequist TD, et al. Differences in the use of telephone and video telemedicine visits during the COVID-19 pandemic. Am J Manag Care 2021;27(1):21–6.

32. Maor E, Tsur N, Barkai G, et al. Noninvasive vocal biomarker is associated with severe acute respiratory syndrome Coronavirus 2 Infection. Mayo Clin Proc Innov Qual Outcomes 2021;5(3):654–62.

Framework for Digital Health Phenotypes in Heart Failure
From Wearable Devices to New Sensor Technologies

Rola Khedraki, MD[a,b], Ajay V. Srivastava, MD[a,b],
Sanjeev P. Bhavnani, MD[a,c],*

KEYWORDS

- Wearable • Digital health • Sensors • Remote Patient monitoring • Analytics
- Clinical decision support

KEY POINTS

- There has been a technological boom in the field of digital health care that includes wearables and sensor-based technologies. This has been brought to the forefront especially in the field of cardiovascular medicine and more specifically in the care of patients with heart failure (HF) cohort with a renewed approach at disease monitoring and risk stratification of the patients with HF.
- Although there continues to be a deluge of software platforms for remote patient monitoring (RPM), clinical trials have offered discrepant results as to whether this strategy truly impacts major outcomes such as HF hospitalizations or cardiovascular mortality as compared with standard of care.
- The HF population is particularly challenging given the high degree of disease heterogeneity, an elderly and aging patient cohort, and the difficulty of fully capturing the overall risk trajectory of the patients with HF with any single data parameter offered by a digital device.
- We propose a new framework of "Digital Phenotypes in HF" for how new devices and sensors and their respective datasets can be leveraged to guide tailored therapy and predict disease progression within this complex patient population to advance HF care delivery.
- We seek to illustrate the patient, technical, and clinical workflow barriers that must be overcome to provide maximum clinical value and provide a framework to properly construct a digital phenotype that aims to risk stratify patients with HF and impact outcomes by leveraging the individualized monitoring and treatment strategies offered by these technologies.

Funding: This work was partially supported by an unrestricted Artificial Intelligence in Imaging educational and research grant sponsored by Scripps Health to S. Bhavnani.

[a] Section of Advanced Heart Failure, Scripps Research Foundation, Scripps Clinic, Prebys Cardiovascular Institute, 9898 Genesee Avenue, AMP-300, La Jolla, CA 920337, USA; [b] Division of Cardiovascular Medicine, Scripps Clinic, Prebys Cardiovascular Institute, 9898 Genesee Avenue, AMP-300, La Jolla, CA 920337, USA; [c] Division of Cardiology, Healthcare Innovation & Practice Transformation Laboratory, Scripps Clinic, Scripps Research Foundation, Prebys Cardiovascular Institute, 9898 Genesee Avenue, AMP-300, La Jolla, CA 920337, USA

* Corresponding author. Division of Cardiology, Healthcare Innovation & Practice Transformation Laboratory, Scripps Clinic, Scripps Research Foundation, Prebys Cardiovascular Institute, 9898 Genesee Avenue, AMP 3-1117, La Jolla, CA 920337.

E-mail address: bhavnani.sanjeev@scripphealth.org

Heart Failure Clin 18 (2022) 223–244
https://doi.org/10.1016/j.hfc.2021.12.003

THE DIGITAL TRANSFORMATION OF HEART FAILURE

The adoption and impact of digital health in heart failure (HF) are rapidly evolving and expanding. This has been driven by the desire on the part of health care providers to capture data that were inaccessible previously within the confines of the traditional practice of medicine. For decades this medical paradigm has defined itself by an episodic model of health care that takes place within the walls of a hospital or clinic.[1,2] The promise of new wearable and digital health technologies to bridge care between visits with a data-driven model of care and improve HF quality metrics including hospitalizations is promising.[3] However, perhaps an even larger momentum for wearables and digital health has come from consumers themselves, with ever-increasing demand and interest among individuals to monitor their own health and progress.[4]

The HF population is a unique cohort in which risk factor identification is paramount in altering the trajectory of a disease in which recurrent hospitalizations have repeatedly been shown to be a strong predictor of mortality.[5] Furthermore, HF medical costs place a considerable strain on the health care system and are projected to be $69.7 billion by 2030.[6,7] Although evidence-based guidelines for medical therapy and interventions exist to prevent or manage HF, a notable treatment gap persists in real-world management with HF being at the forefront of hospitalizations among older adults.[6,8] Of the many challenges with managing HF effectively is the prediction of imminent decompensation[9] and to identify, risk-stratify, and optimally treat[10] at-risk individuals with HF at risk for future morbidity and mortality. Studies using implantable devices to monitor the pathophysiologic changes that occur in the transition from compensated to a congested state have shown that changes in weight and symptoms are in fact late findings.[11] Therefore, the ability to use digital tools to augment the collection of more granular data to identify patients in a hemodynamically stable and presymptomatic congestion phase is essential to preventing hospitalizations, and thereby impacting prognosis.[12] Undoubtedly, the coronavirus disease-2019 (COVID-19) pandemic has forced the medical community to review current clinical practices and has provided the impetus for the rapid digitization of medicine and telehealth toward virtual and remote care.[13]

Digital Health and Wearable Technologies

There are several classifications of digital technologies that can be considered for patient monitoring. Such technologies include wearable and wireless devices (patch-based devices), smartphone-connected technologies (single/multiple-lead ECG, handheld ultrasound, blood pressure, and glucose monitoring devices), implantable sensors (pulmonary artery sensors, continuous glucose monitoring), and various lab-on-a-chip platforms.[1] Wearable technologies are one classification of digital devices and are commonly defined as those devices that capture functional and physiologic data such as actigraphy, sleep monitors, and smart clothing, and those that are commercially available, procured by consumers for self-monitoring, and are used by individuals in their daily living with findings that are not commonly conveyed to clinicians for medical decisions[14] (**Fig. 1**). These digital devices are constantly expanding and becoming increasingly sophisticated in their ability to quantify physiologic measurements through advanced computational approaches, thus challenging our contemporary methods for how risk is measured and ultimately for how HF is detected and monitored. In the context of HF, we can elucidate an important differentiation with such devices. For example, the association between smartphone-connected devices such as blood pressure, glucometry, and ECG devices are well suited for monitoring hypertension, diabetes, and arrhythmias, respectively, as the device measurements are the same measurements that can be modified with lifestyle and pharmacotherapy. In contrast, digital health devices in HF are heterogeneous with no single wearable device (activity, sleep, heart rate, blood pressure, or weight) capturing sufficient information on which a treatment strategy can be created. Thus, the need for a systematic approach to evaluation and validation is required, and to consider pragmatic approaches for unique HF cohorts.[15] For simplicity and to discuss the potential applications of new devices in HF, we will refer to "digital health" that includes wearable devices and sensor-based technologies as they apply to various aspects of remote monitoring, care delivery, and for patient–clinician communications.

THE HYPOTHESIS OF BENEFIT WITH WEARABLE AND DIGITAL HEALTH DEVICES IN HEART FAILURE

There is a widely accepted hypothesis that digital health, including wearables, as part of RPM among patients with HF can be beneficial. While this hypothesis continues to be the impetus for the development of clinical programs for HF management, the results from large randomized clinical trials have demonstrated conflicting results

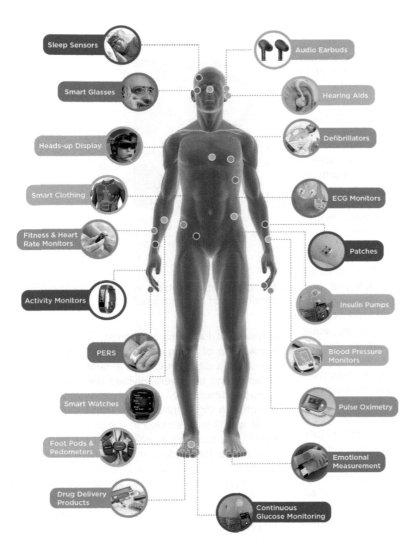

Fig. 1. Variety of wearable and digital health devices that are currently available or under development. PERS, Personal Emergency Response System.

with no difference in major outcomes of HF-related hospitalization or cardiovascular mortality compared with standard, conventional HF practices without the use of digital devices.[16–18] Furthermore, the aggregate of randomized trials has demonstrated significant heterogeneity that is largely attributable to factors ranging from the baseline risk of patients monitored (those with or without a preceding HF hospitalization) and the type of digital health devices used (single biometric measurements such as weight vs multiparametric monitoring with multiple devices), to how patient-generated data were monitored by clinical staff and with what frequency clinical decisions were made (ie, daily, weekly, or monthly).[19] We suggest the following explanations for the discordance between the anticipated clinical utility and the lack of uniform benefit from randomized trials:

- The same monitoring strategy using the same suite of devices does not apply equally across patients with HF and among whom baseline risk dictates the time to or recurrence of an HF outcome.
- HF is a heterogeneous condition with variability in the underlying pathophysiology; therefore, while surrogate biomarkers markers of cardiac function such as actigraphy, blood pressure, HR, heart rhythm, and weight are predictive of outcomes in HF, they are not modifiable to the degree necessary to prevent such outcomes. In parallel, the time horizon required to change these biometrics may not be the same as the time duration of remote monitoring (ie, 3 months, 6 months, 12 months, etc.).
- Substrate monitoring, in contrast to surrogate biomarkers, with new sensors such as

wearable electro-mechanical PPG devices and Tissue Doppler imaging technologies may yield more precise datasets toward measuring myocardial function and detecting changes in the remodeled left ventricle.

- Digital health datasets derived from remote monitoring are not commonly analyzed in parallel to a given patient's breadth of electronic medical record (EMR) data. This can include laboratory results, imaging, ECG, echocardiography, or non-EMR data such as pharmacy data (ie, medication compliance or adverse side effects resulting from polypharmacy). Therefore, the data captured from remote monitoring alone may not sufficiently capture HF-related risk.

If we aim to make digital health a standard for HF care, it first requires an understanding of how patient-related factors and device utilization intersect to more precisely identify patient-level risk, and how technology and data-driven processes advance toward individualized strategies for HF-monitoring.[1] We propose a new framework—Digital Phenotypes in HF—that aims to determine which type of technology is best used in which patients with HF and how the derived datasets can be used predict disease trajectory and to enable continuous patient participation within the HF process of care. Within this framework, we can join the following 4 synergistic priorities to form the foundation on which digital health devices can advance care delivery: (1) Develop a codesigned, patient-centered digital health strategy within the continuity of HF-related care; (2) implement digital health technologies and new sensors within remote patient monitoring (RPM) programs centered on patient-generated data; (3) understand digital phenotyping and the computational methods necessary to produce individualized approaches to risk assessments and treatments in HF; and (4) us dynamic clinical decision support systems that integrate digital health, remote monitoring data with EMRs, and how such data are translated to population health HF programs. Developing a systematic approach that incorporates HF digital phenotypes with these synergies will best position our efforts to answer the aforementioned questions, offer exposition to the above-stated explanations, and ultimately to test our hypothesis (**Fig. 2**).

Digital Phenotypes in Heart Failure

The concept of digital phenotyping refers to the in situ quantification of an individual's biometric and behavioral data with the objective of exploiting this data to offer a direct measure or proxy for

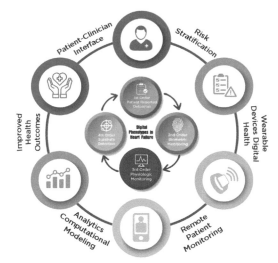

Fig. 2. Digital phenotypes in heart failure within the continuum of healthcare delivery.

physiologic functions of interest.[20–22] The clinical application of being equipped with the ability to construct a digital map is an essential component of achieving truly personalized care in an era of precision medicine. Although the idea of constructing a digital phenotype using digital health tools was first described in the psychiatric literature,[21] this concept is well poised for its application to the longitudinal management of HF. We advocate for using a novel schematic for digital phenotypes as it relates to HF to build markers and harness raw data to predict clinical outcomes. Herein, we have characterized 4 subtypes of digital phenotypes in HF:

First-order digital phenotype: Patient-generated data such as patient-reported outcomes (PROs) collected on an app-based platform for longitudinal assessments of symptoms and quality of life.

Second-order digital phenotype: Biometric monitoring with wearable and digital health devices such as activity, blood pressure, heart rate and rhythm, and weight monitoring devices within RPM programs.

Third-order digital phenotype: Physiologic monitoring at the cardio-pulmonary level with implantable cardiac devices and sensor-based technologies.

Fourth-order digital phenotype: Substrate detection with newly developed wearable and digital technologies for continuous intracardiac pressure measurements and for the prediction of contractile dysfunction.

It is our objective to use these 4 subtypes within a construct of remote monitoring that applies to the continuum between digital devices, patients, and clinicians, and illustrate how such digital phenotypes apply to patients with HF through an appraisal of the literature (**Table 1**) and real-world evidence examples.

DIGITAL HEALTH— PATIENT CODESIGNS AND PARTICIPATORY MODELS OF HEART FAILURE CARE

Before considering digital devices for patient care it is important to appreciate how a participatory model is leveraged for optimal utilization. A technology acceptance model is a framework that models how users come to accept and use a new technology. Technology acceptance models based on the "Theory of Reasoned Action"—which explains the relationship between human attitudes and behaviors—state that key factors for new technology adoption in patient care are its perceived ease of use and usefulness.[23] The key components for technology acceptance that are important for patients are fundamentally rooted within core principals of adoption, which include (1) identifying the determinants of adoption at the individual level (ie, functionality and operational efficiency), (2) testing the proposed adoption (ie, how digital information flows between the patient, caregiver, and clinician), and (3) developing a pre and postimplementation strategy that can enhance a patient's use of a new technology (ie, iterative testing with user feedback). New technology models, particularly for those with chronic conditions, harness "co-designs," in which patients and the clinical team design a technology strategy that includes mutual acceptance of the type of device selected, its experience, and its expectations toward improving health literacy and health management skills.[24] While we advocate for an upfront strategy that includes such systematic approaches before the utilization of new digital technologies, there exist significant barriers to digital health uptake particularly in older adults who commonly face unique physical or cognitive challenges with adapting to technology workflows and developing confidence in using digital tools. As a result, there has been an increased focus on the development of geriatric-sensitive technology that aims to close the gap between older adults and the technological tools designed to serve them.[25,26]

Only by understanding the current state of the field can we create actionable initiatives that too often assume patient participation but lacks sound evidence to become effective in engaging patient and caregiver participation.[1] This digital health translational gap in integrating health technologies into their respective clinical applications can only be adequately addressed when backed by evidence for benefit with regards to patient management or outcomes in a clinically important and patient-centric manner.[27] A simple example would be smartphone technology, which has become more mainstream, which can be an attractive platform in anticipating a new smartphone-based technology as having broad applications to an HF population. However, a digital divide still exists within the confines of social determinants of health and socioeconomic and geographic barriers that impede participation in real-world application of these programs.[28] This digital divide in the HF population was highlighted by Pezel and colleagues, who surveyed nearly 3000 patients with chronic HF to evaluate the use of smartphones and feasibility of using this technology for health care delivery.[29] The authors found that 36% of patients were smartphone users and that these patients tended to be younger, male, lived in cities, had higher educational level, and more frequently held positions such as company executives and independent professionals than patients without a smartphone. Furthermore, only 22% of patients were actively participating in a therapeutic educational program but that those with smartphones were more observant with maintaining low sodium diets and frequently weighing themselves even after adjusting for multiple confounding factors. Although the study was conducted within a community cohort at their health care system, and therefore not generalizable to the broader HF community, the results are nonetheless telling of the importance of thoroughly evaluating the population of interest and gauging the acceptance of a technology program before implementation.

FIRST-ORDER DIGITAL PHENOTYPE—APP-BASED PATIENT-GENERATED HEALTH DATA AND PATIENT-REPORTED OUTCOMES

The first-order digital phenotype in HF management is derived from patient-generated health data (PGHD) derived from PROs. This relies on patient engagement and patient data entry into smartphone app-based technology including, among others, self-reported symptoms, diet, weight, mood, sleep quality, medication compliance[19,30] (**Fig. 3**). This is particularly relevant in the present day whereby there are nearly 350,000 "health apps" that are available to patients and their caregivers.[31] The value of tracking PROs in an HF population is multifaceted. First, this practice empowers patients by making them the owners of their data and how they choose to connect to and engage with their health care providers.[32] Second, it leads to increased awareness

Table 1
List of key studies involving digital health devices in patients with HF according to digital phenotype

Author, year, Study Name	Aim	Digital Phenotype Leveraged	Trial design	Population	Sample size	Primary Outcome	Main Findings
First Order Digital Phenotype							
Bakogiannis et al,[73] 2021	Patient, physician, caregiver co development of a smartphone- app for HF usability assessment and quality of life measures	First order (QoL)	Prospective usability study to investigate the effect of app use among patients with HF	Patients with ambulatory HF	App development from 18 app features	Quality of life metrics	Trend toward increase in mean quality of life after 3 mo according to KCCQ (mean increase 5.8 [SD 15] points, 95% CI -0.1–11.6, P = .054) and EQ-5D-5 L (mean increase 5.6% [SD 15.6%], 95% CI -0.4–11.5, P = .06).
ThessHF					Usability study: 14 patients Pilot study: 30 patients	(KCCQ) 5-level EQ-5D	Increase in quality of self-care by 4.4% (SD 7.2%, 95% CI 1.7–7.1, P = .002) according to the European Heart Failure Self-care Behavior Scale (secondary outcome)
Dwinger et al,[74] 2020	Evaluate the effectiveness of telephone based health coaching (TBHC) on patient-reported outcomes and health behaviors	First-order (PRO) + Telephone Health Coaching	Prospective, RCT TBHC intervention vs usual care TBHC comprised of Daily vital sign self-monitoring and weekly telehealth video visits	Patients with ≥1 chronic conditions	4283	Effects of TBHC on QOL and health behaviors	TBHC was superior to control group in 6 of 19 outcomes including weekly physical activity (P = .03), metabolic rate per week (P = .048), BMI (P = .009), self-monitoring blood pressure (P < .001), patient activation (P < .001), and measures of health literacy (P < .001)
Pekmezaris et al,[75] 2019	To compare utilization and QOL for underserved black and Hispanic HF patients assigned to telehealth self-monitoring (TSM)	First-order (PRO) + QoL + Telehealth	Prospective RCT	Underserved black and Hispanic patients within 72 h from HF hospitalization discharge and NYHA I-II symptoms	104	Inpatient and ED utilization QOL (MHHFQ) (PHQ-4)	TSM was not effective in meeting the primary endpoints for underserved patients with HF: ED visits (RR 1.37, CI 0.83–2.27) Hospitalization (RR 0.92, CI 0.57–1.48) Length of Stay (0.54 vs 0.91 d) No differences in QOL between groups over 90 d (P = .5)

	Aim	Digital Phenotype	Study design	Population	N	Outcome measure	Results
Goldstein et al,[76] 2014	Feasibility of using an electronic pill box and smartphone-based app intervention to improve medication adherence in patients with HF over 28 d	First-order (PRO) + Medication Adherence Smartphone App	Prospective RCT 4 groups: smartphone silent, smartphone reminding, pillbox silent, pillbox reminding	Age 45–90 with NYHA class II-III for Ambulatory patients with HFrEF EF <40%	60	Medication adherence	Overall adherence rate of 78%. Electronic pill box adherence rate 80% of the time vs, smartphone app 76% of the time (no difference in adherence rate whether patients were given a reminder)
Second Order Digital Phenotype							
Redfield et al,[77] 2015 NEAT-HFpEF	To evaluate the effect of isosorbide mononitrate on daily activity in patients with HF as assessed by patient-worn accelerometers	Second-order (actigraphy)	Multicenter RCT, double-blind, placebo-controlled, crossover study: 1:1 assignment to one of the 2 treatment groups (6 wk of placebo with crossover to 6 wk of isosorbide mononitrate vs 6 wk of isosorbide mononitrate with crossover to 6 wk of placebo	Ambulatory patients with HFpEF with EF $\geq$ 50%	110	Average daily accelerometer units during period in which patients receiving a target dose of 120 mg of isosorbide mononitrate were compared to placebo	Trend toward lower daily activity in patients receiving the 120 mg dose of isosorbide mononitrate (-381 accelerometer units; CI - 780-17, $P = .06$) and a significant decrease in hours of activity per day (-0.30 h; CI $= 0.55$ to -0.05, $P = .02$). During all dose regimens, activity in the isosorbide mononitrate group was lower than placebo and there were no significant between- group differences in 6MWT, QOL, or NT pro- BNP levels (secondary endpoints)
Koehler et al,[78] 2011 TIM-HF	Investigate the impact of dedicated telemedical management on mortality in patients with ambulatory CHF	First-order (PROs) Second- order (EKG, BP weight monitoring)	Prospective RCT, 1:1	NYHA II/III, LVEF $\leq$35%, Prior HF hospitalization within 24 mo	710	All-cause mortality CV mortality HF hospitalization	Compared to usual care, remote telemedical management was not associated with reduction in all-cause mortality (HR 0.97, CI 0.67–1.41, $P = .87$), or CV death or HF hospitalization (HR 0.89, CI 0.67–1.19, $P = .44$)

(continued on next page)

Table 1
(continued)

Author, year, Study Name	Aim	Digital Phenotype Leveraged	Trial design	Population	Sample size	Primary Outcome	Main Findings
Koehler et al,[16] 2018	Investigate the efficacy of remote patient management plus usual care vs usual care alone in patients with ambulatory CHF	First-order (PROs)	Prospective RCT, 1:1	NYHA II/III LVEF ≤ 45%	1571	Percentage of days lost due to unplanned cardiovascular hospital admissions or all-cause death	Percent of days lost due to unplanned cardiovascular admission and all-cause death were 4.88% (CI 4.55–5.23) in the remote monitoring group vs 6.64% (CI 6.19–7.13) in the usual care group (ratio 0.80, CI 0.65–1.00, P = .0460).
TIM-HF2		Second-order (EKG, BP)		Prior HF hospitalization within 12			No significant difference in cardiovascular mortality between groups (secondary endpoint); HR 0.671, CI 0.45–1.01, P = .0560.
Ong et al,[79] 2016 BEAT-HF	Evaluate the effectiveness of RPM in reducing readmissions among adults hospitalized with HF	First-order (PROs) Second-order (EKG, BP, weight, oximetry)	Prospective RCT, 1:1	NYHA III/IV ADHF Hospitalized patients with HF Any LVEF (mean LVEF 43%)	1437	Readmission for any cause within 180 d after discharge	Among patients hospitalized for HF, combined health coaching telephone calls and telemonitoring did not reduce 180-d readmissions which occurred in 50.8% and 49.2% of patients in the intervention and usual care groups, respectively (adjusted hazard ratio, 1.03; 95% CI, 0.88–1.20; P = .74).

Study/Device	Objective	Technology	Study Design	Population	N	Outcomes	Results
Clays et al,[80] 2021 HeartMan	Evaluate the effectiveness of HeartMan, a smartphone app which is connected to several sensing devices including a custom wristband and cloud service	First-order (PRO Mental and Sexual Health) + Second- order (BP, smart pill organizer, wrist band measuring heart rate variability, skin galvanic response, temperature, and acceleration)	Randomized proof of concept trial (1:2 ratio of control: intervention)	Patients with ambulatory HF	56	Health related QOL (HRQoL), and self-management	Compared to control, reduction in depression and anxiety in intervention group (P < .001). Non-significant improvements in self-care (P < .05) and decrease in sexual problems (P < .05) in the intervention group. Significant reduction in need for sexual counseling in the control group (P < .05). No significant effect on HRQoL, self-care confidence, illness perception, exercise capacity (6MWT)
Third Order Digital Phenotype							
Amir et al,[81] 2017 ReDS	To evaluate the feasibility of using ReDS-directed fluid management to reduce HF readmissions	Dielectric Properties of Lung Fluid content	Prospective, observational study	Any patients with LVEF screened during an index ADHF event	50	HF readmission Study endpoints were collected during the ReDS-guided management as well as 3 mo pre and poststudy for comparison	The readmission rate during the ReDS-guided management period was 0.04 events/patient/3 mo as compared to the pre and post-ReDS readmission rates of 0.3 and 0.19 events/patient/3 mo, respectively. ReDS-guided management led to an 87% reduction in admission compared to the pre- ReDS period and 79% reduction compared to the post-ReDS period
Lala et al,[82] 2021 ReDS	To evaluate whether the use of ReDS would lower 30-d readmission	Dielectric Properties of Lung Fluid content	Retrospective observational cohort study	All patients discharged after an HF admission within 10 d of discharge	220 (ReDS performed in 80)	30-d CV and all-cause hospital readmission after index HF hospitalization	ReDS use led to reduction in 30-d CV readmission (2.6% vs 11.8%, HR 0.21, CI 0.05–0.89, P = .04) and trend toward decrease in all-cause readmission (6.5% vs 14.1%, HR 0.43, CI 0.16–1.15, P = .09)

(continued on next page)

Table 1
(continued)

Fourth Order Digital Phenotype

Author, year, Study Name	Aim	Digital Phenotype Leveraged	Trial design	Population	Sample size	Primary Outcome	Main Findings
Inan et al,[83] 2018	To evaluate HF state by measuring electrical and mechanical function with a wearable ECG and a seismocardio gram patch	Ballistocardiogram Seismocardiography (SCG) + Machine Learning analysis on continuous, time-series dataset	Prospective, observational study	Ambulatory and hospitalized HF patients	45	Quantification of the spectral domain similarity between the measured SCG signal as a surrogate of cardiovascular hemodynamics and cardiac contractility before and after 6MWT	Graph similarity scores were significantly higher for the decompensated vs compensated patients: 44.4 ± 4.9 vs 35.2 ± 10.6, $P < .01$, implying SCG prediction for HF decompensation A significant change in GSS from admission to discharge was observed in 6 decompensated patients with longitudinal data, 44 ± 4.1 (admitted) vs 35 ± 3.9 (discharged), $P < .05$.
					13 ADHF, 32 patients with ambulatory HF		
Liu et al 2021,[84]	Opto- mechanical system to measure non-invasive and automatic continuous blood pressure (CBP)	Capillary Blood Pressure	Prospective, observational study	Four categories: 1. patients with no CV disease 2. patients with PAD 3. patients with varicose veins 4. patients with HF	40	Response of CBP measurements results to subject categories	A noninvasive CBP system can track local CBP changes induced by different levels of venous congestion and could classify HF patients with an AUC of 0.90.

| Shah et al,[85] 2020 | To evaluate whether wristband technologies may facilitate more accurate bedside testing | Photoplethysmography + Accelerometry | Proof of concept cross-sectional analysis. | Wristband to capture PPG and 3-axis accelerometry measured at rest and while doing 5 valsalva maneuvers over 1 min. Extracted 4 features of beat-to-beat variability and signal quality which were used as inputs to a machine learned classification algorithm | 97 (54 patients with HF) | ADHF | Patients recruited at random from an inpatient sample of patients admitted for CAD, HF, or arrhythmia management | The waveform-based features alone achieved an AUC of 0.8 with an overall accuracy of 74%. When a sensitivity threshold of 90% was used, the specificity was 50%. When demographics, medical history and vital signs were included the AUC improved to 0.87 and specificity to 72%. AUC for the model in HFrEF vs no HF was 0.92, and for HFpEF vs no HF was 0.85. |

Refs. [16,73–85]

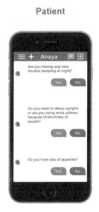

Patient

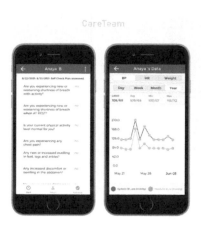

CareTeam

Fig. 3. 1st order digital phenotype Example of patient generated health data (PGHD) and patient-reported outcomes (PROs) in HF. collected on a smartphone health application for review by patients and clinical teams.

of health and enables patients to become active participants in their own wellness.[32] Third, it allows patients to gain a deeper understanding of the important trends that inform management decisions from their treatment team, and consequently, helps patients understand when to seek care.[32] Having active engagement from patients with HF is an essential part of being able to support this patient population. There are many strategies of incentivizing patients to maintain engagement and support retention including gamification-enabled applications and connectivity to social support communities through these app-based technologies.[32]

Although there lies much potential in tracking PROs, there are also many challenges. A study evaluating the effectiveness of 10 apps to improve HF self-care evaluated app functionality using the 11-item IMS Institute for Healthcare Informatics app functionality scoring system found that most of the apps evaluated performed well with 9 out of 10 achieving a score greater than 8 with higher scores reflecting a more comprehensive app.[33] However, app functionality does not necessarily translate to benefit in outcomes and, as the authors note, the greatest barrier to the uptake of health apps continues to be the lack of evidence demonstrating value.[34] A systematic review evaluating the impact of app-based HF management interventions found highly inconsistent outcomes with regards to all-cause mortality, cardiovascular mortality, HF-related hospitalizations, length of stay, NYHA functional class, LVEF, quality of life, and self-care.[33,35] Furthermore, the studies analyzed demonstrated rates of high attrition and limited long-term engagement. These results highlight a fundamental problem with app-based care and further complicate the ability to determine whether a lack of effectiveness is related to poor

patient adherence or ineffective digital engagement.[36] In the context of medication adherence with smartphone-medication compliance apps, several models of care are currently underway to address patient engagement for long-term utilization including: text-messaging[37] to target medication adherence; behavioral messaging to promote lifestyle changes that are disease specific[38] (hypertension, atrial fibrillation, coronary disease, or HF) to encourage patient participation along the trajectory of their underlying condition; and an interdisciplinary pharmacist driven program that combines medication adherence from pharmacy data with important PROs of quality of life and to track both over time.[39]

SECOND-ORDER DIGITAL PHENOTYPE—DIGITAL DEVICE BIOMETRIC MONITORING

The second-order digital phenotype in HF refers to biometric monitoring which can link RPM vital sign data and anthropometric measures with PGHD (**Fig. 4**A–C). This includes the integration of patient inputted data from the first-order digital phenotype with multiple digital devices including smartphone-connected devices (blood pressure, glucose levels, and weight), activity monitoring (daily step count and gait speed), smartphone-connected ECG, and consumer-based wearable devices such as sleep monitors and mood tracking technologies for psychological wellbeing.[40] On one hand, a multitude of devices are available for any given patients with HF that enables the tracking of multiple biometric measures necessary to understand the variability in signs and symptoms including monitoring changes in recorded weights, detection of increased usage of diuretic via a "smart" pill box, changes in sleep or activity patterns,[41] and impedance markers of fluid

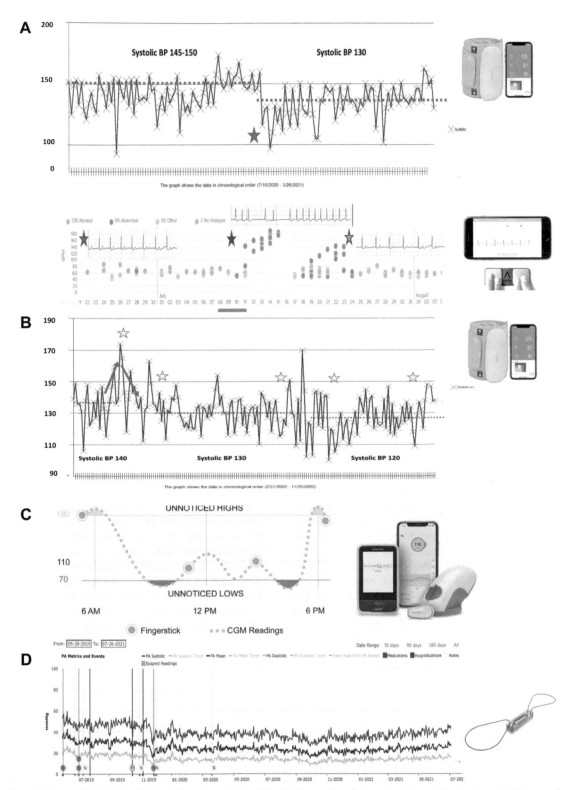

Fig. 4. 2nd and 3rd Order Digital Phenotypes: Real-World Examples of Remote Patient Monitoring in HF. In each scenario, all care coordination was performed virtually with no face-to-face encounters. (*A*): Home-based blood pressure monitoring in a 68-year old man with ischemic cardiomyopathy, HFrEF (EF 25%) with recovery (EF 55%), obesity (BMI 45) on multiple antihypertensive therapies. Began intermittent fasting (blue star) resulting in an

overload.[14] On the other, we must consider various patients, technical, and clinical workflow-related factors for using multiple devices on a frequent basis over a long period of engagement[1] (**Table 2**). Both aspects must be taken together within an evolving model of health care data aggregation that may be particularly applicable for an elderly cohort with HF, or those more advanced states of LV dysfunction.[42]

If we are to consider new wearable devices and those that are increasingly commercially available, then we must first consider the lessons learned from digital health devices used in HF.[19,30] While there are many reasons for the lack of uniform benefit from randomized clinical trials in HF using digital health biometric monitoring devices, the heterogeneity among patients with HF is a fundamental reason. This can be seen within the same HF classification (HFrEF or HFpEF) for which the variability can be extensive as the underlying pathophysiology is multifactorial (ischemic vs nonischemic), and the response to changes in preload and/or afterload are variable at the anatomic (valvular regurgitation/stenosis), and functional levels (increases in left ventricular, left atrial, and pulmonary venous/arterial pressures). In the aggregate, these variables can result in a differential risk of outcomes such as ischemia, progressive LV dysfunction, and arrhythmias.[43,44] The challenge between biometric monitoring and the heterogeneity within HF cohorts can be further explained by taking 3 of the large RPM trials into discussion. The TIM-HF[17] and TIM-HF2[16] (Telemedical Interventional Monitoring in Heart Failure) and the BEAT-HF[18] (Better Effectiveness After Transition—Heart Failure) trials that randomized stable ambulatory patients with HF with a prior HF hospitalization in the previous 24 months (TIM-HF; EF <35%, NYHA II–III); ambulatory patients with HF with a prior hospitalization in the previous 12 months (TIM-HF2; EF<45%, NYHA II–III); and patients with ADHF immediately before hospital discharge (BEAT-HF; any LVEF [mean EF 43%], NYHA III–IV). Compared with standard care, over a follow-up duration of 6 months (BEAT-HF), 12 months (TIM-HF2), and 26 months (TIM-HF), RPM with digital health devices including weight, blood pressure, ECG, and/or oximetry did not demonstrate a difference in outcomes of HF hospitalization or CV-mortality in the TIM-HF or BEAT-HF studies; however, did result in a reduction in all-cause hospitalizations and all-cause mortality in the TIM-HF2 study (see **Table 1**). From these results, one can ascertain that a standardized approach to RPM with the same type of devices across different cohorts of patients with HF with variable baseline risk for outcomes is not effective and that the underlying heterogeneity in cardiac function cannot be accurately measured with surrogate biomarkers, or measured equally, across HF cohorts with varying severity of the disease.[45,46]

Applying transitive properties of equality, in that, if we equate new wearable devices with digital health technologies, then we must consider the type of patients with HF, the type of technologies used for monitoring and, parallel, the HF outcomes of interest. Wearable devices such as activity monitors, sleep monitors, smartwatches, clothing embedded with sensors, and other commercially available technologies have yet to be sufficiently validated through robust clinical trials, postmarket surveillance, or real-world evidence programs.[2,14] As such we are challenged to understand how to align datasets such as sleep quantity/quality, activity, gait speed, and mood disturbances such as depression, which are dynamic and changing within patients with HF, with what type of outcomes they should be measured against.[47] While it is possible that sleep quality may have an impact on outcomes such as HF hospitalization, we would not expect an association with outcomes of mortality, HF, CV, or otherwise. Given the variability in outcomes from vital sign monitoring digital devices, questions arise if wearable technologies themselves acquire the correct measurements or

improvement in BP control. (*B*): Smartphone-ECG and home-based BP monitoring in a 74-year old with persistent AF, NICM (EF 25%) due to tachycardia-mediated cardiomyopathy. Underwent AF ablation (blue star), recurrence of rapid AF and initiation of antiarrhythmic therapy with amiodarone (red star), and repeat AF ablation (green star) to sinus rhythm. Titration of GDMT with metoprolol, sacubitril-valsartan, spironolactone, and dapagliflozin (yellow stars) with improvements in afterload reduction. (*C*) Continuous glucose monitoring in a 64-year old with type-2 diabetes, ischemic heart disease, and HF with mid-range EF (45%). Observations of AM and PM hypoglycemia that required adjustments in medical therapies to prevent further hypoglycemic episodes. (*D*) Pulmonary artery sensor guided therapy in a 70-year old with HFrEF (EF 20%) due to ischemic cardiomyopathy. Implantation after an HF hospitalization (2019) with medication titration based on PA pressures (orange and yellow *lines*) resulting in rapid reduction in PA systolic pressure from 60 mm Hg to less than 40 mm Hg and sustained throughout 2020 to 2021. Parallel improvements in dyspnea and orthopnea as well as improvements in QoL were observed.

Table 2
Key considerations for wearable and digital health device utilization by patients and clinicians

Digital Health Consideration	Description
Patient-Related Considerations	
Digital Literacy	The baseline familiarity with common digital technologies such as smartphones, computers, tables, and Internet usage
Digital Retention	Determinants of longitudinal and persistent utilization of a smartphone health application, wearable, or digital health device
Digital Engagement	Mechanisms to increase engagement with a digital technology that can include caregiver participation, community-networks, social media, and text- messaging
Digital Access	Understand socio-economic barriers to acquiring digital health technologies, Broadband/WIFI availability, cultural and linguistic sensitive approaches for patient education and engagement
Physical and Cognitive Limitations	Motor skills, hand–eye coordination, time to complete digital tasks, visual and auditory acuity, processing speed, attention, and recollection
Device-Related Considerations	
Privacy Concerns	Align the requirements for digital health devices utilization with personal preferences with privacy and security
Cost of Acquisition	Determine the most streamlined method for device procurement including patient purchase, health savings accounts, insurance coverage, local/federal programs, clinic purchase, no-cost options
Active vs Passive Monitoring	Active denotes patient participation and performing various tasks on digital platforms vs passive implying no touch, continuous data acquisition sensors that do not require patient participation
Interoperability	Determine the optimal mechanisms for integrating multiple digital health devices on a single digital platform
Device Designs and Form Factor	Understand how a given user interfaces with a digital tool, size of the device, various device operations, charging, visual dashboards
Meaningful and Modifiable Signal	For a given patient with HF the type of measurement acquired must be clinically relevant to both the patient and the clinician for how it is modified to improve symptoms and quality of life
Clinical Workflow-Related Considerations	
Clinical Decision Support	Develop clinical decision support tools as part of remote monitoring and to determine individualized treatment strategies
Clinical Workflows	Ensure clinical teams understand the application of digital health for HF monitoring
Data Overload	Balance the large volume of remotely monitored data (intermittent and continuous) with the frequency of follow-up
Balance between disease tracking and tie horizon for monitoring	Determine the optimal time duration for monitoring (1, 3, 6, 12 mo) based on baseline HF risk and the risk of HF outcomes such as hospital readmissions.

measurements that are modified to the degree necessary to improve major outcomes of morbidity or mortality. In contrast, first-order phenotypes and health-related quality-of-life (QoL) measures are powerful assessments of a health condition coming directly from patients on their perceptions, feelings, and functional limitations that spans psychometric and emotional, to social and activities of daily living.[48] In this context, wearable devices may be optimally positioned and aligns the type of device with a patient's main QoL limitation to generate individualized monitoring strategies at the per patient level. Recent data from HF telerehabilitation clinical trials[49,50] have demonstrated an association between a monitoring strategy with wearable devices and the assessments of QoL (Kansas City Cardiomyopathy Questionnaire), sleep (Spiegel Sleep Questionnaire), and general health and social function (Medical Outcome Survey Short Form-36) with results that suggest PROs are a viable tool to marry RPM with those symptoms most important to a given patient. Presently, while such approaches remain theoretic, the data toward their efficacy with wearable technologies in HF are promising.

THIRD-ORDER DIGITAL PHENOTYPE— IMPLANTABLE SENSORS FOR PHYSIOLOGIC MONITORING

The third-order digital phenotype refers to implantable devices for which there has been much development in the HF arena. Perhaps the most noteworthy has been the CardioMEMS (Abbott, Sylmar, CA), a monitoring system that remotely measures pulmonary artery pressures (PAPs) via a sensor in the pulmonary artery[51] (**Fig. 4**D). In the landmark CHAMPION trial,[51] PAP-guided therapy in patients with NYHA class III symptoms and ≥ 1 HF hospitalization in the past 12 months led to a 28% reduction of HF hospitalization in the treatment group at 6 months (hazard ratio (HR): 0.72, 95% confidence interval (CI): 0.60–0.85, $P = .0002$) and by 37% (HR: 0.63, 95% CI: 0.52–0.77, $P < .0001$) over the study period (mean of 15 months).

A follow-up observational study[52] evaluating the real-world effectiveness of CardioMEMS evaluated the first consecutive 2000 patients implanted with several intriguing results: (1) Patient compliance was excellent with an average of 1.2 days between remote pressure transmissions. (2) Adherence in older patients was superior to younger subjects, highlighting the unique ability of this technology to be synergistic with an older cohort. (3) 34% of patients had HFpEF, an HF population that has been characteristically challenging to show improved outcomes.

The favorable results of the CHAMPION trial as well as postmarketing studies[51–56] continue to generate a great deal of enthusiasm for exploring expanded populations that may benefit from this technology. The GUIDE HF trial is a prospective trial that aims to evaluate remote PAP monitoring in a broader cohort with NYHA class II–IV symptoms. CardioMEMS has also been shown as an effective strategy for monitoring changes in PAP and metrics of right ventricular (RV) function, suggesting potential value for risk assessment and titration of PAH medications.[57] In a small observational study,[58] CardioMEMS monitoring in patients undergoing optimization before LVAD surgery helped stratify those with mean PAP greater than 25 mm Hg as higher risk for the combined end point of all-cause mortality, renal complications, and RV failure providing promise for remote tailoring of pump settings.

The CardioMEMS device has created a blueprint for remote hemodynamic profiling for the construction of a third-order digital phenotype and offers advantages as compared with alternative implantable data sources including surrogate markers of fluid accumulation such as thoracic impedance[59–63] or the HeartLogic algorithm (data from multiple sensors to capture heart sounds, transthoracic impedance, respiration, activity, and heart rate),[64–66] which lack evidence for consistently providing actionable data. This highlights the importance of appraising devices and algorithms by applying systematic scientific rigor to validate their utility in the population of interest.

FOURTH-ORDER DIGITAL PHENOTYPE—SUBSTRATE DETECTION

On the horizon are next-generation digital health devices including new wearable technologies that capture multidimensional datasets of continuous physiologic and cardiovascular parameters. If we postulate that no 2 patients with HF have the same outcome despite similar biometric measurements due to variability in the underlying physiologic state, then we are tasked with understanding and monitoring cardiac function at the individual level.[67] New wearable biosensors (**Fig. 5**A) have been recently developed that acquire high dimensional data sets recorded at high frequencies. These datasets aggregate measurements collected simultaneously such as heart rate, heart rate variability, respiratory rate, oxygen saturation, pulse wave, skin temperature, biogalvanic currents, and actigraphy in a single device[68] worn for 23-h a day. In a 24-person feasibility study (mean age 89 years) recording nearly 250,000 person hours of data, simultaneous capture of PGHD and multidimensional datasets produced a timestamp for trends in data before, during and after the onset of a PRO (**Fig. 5**B). Using computational modelings such as machine learning and convolution neural networks in a continuous, time-series dataset enabled the development of predictive models for the occurrence of symptoms including symptomatic HF for individualized N-of-1 monitoring.[69]

Advances in signal transduction technology and the miniaturization of ultrasound devices to piezoelectric nanosensors are under development and in transcutaneous, wearable, and conformable configurations (**Fig. 5**C). Xu and colleagues[70] recently demonstrated a prototype of an "ultrasonic phased array" nanosensor for active beam-steering hemodynamic monitoring at a tissue depth of 3 to 14 cm (see **Fig. 5**C). In a proof-of-concept study, the ultrathin (240 μm) piezoelectric sensor captured 2D-Doppler and tissue Doppler spectra to quantify the directionality of blood flow and ventricular/annual wall motion of cardiac time intervals (iso-volumetric contraction and ejection duration) in real-time, respectively, with an accuracy that was comparable to commercial ultrasound devices. As we await future validation studies, these developments in nanotechnologies with stretchable, skin-based microfabrication enable noninvasive, continuous monitoring of cardiovascular physiology including blood flow, cardiac output, and arterial blood pressure from multiple body locations for potential application to HF remote hemodynamic monitoring.

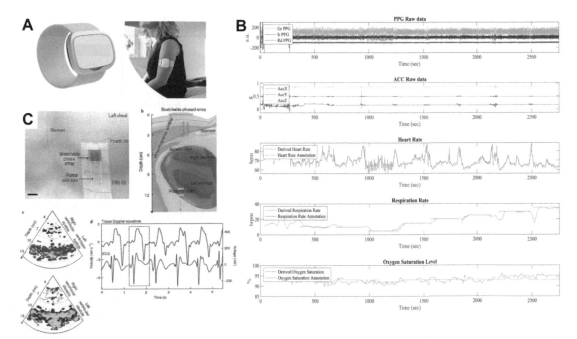

Fig. 5. Examples of 4th Order Digital Phenotypes and Devices for Substrate Monitoring. (*A*) A wearable device for multidimensional physiologic monitoring generating continuous time series datasets (*B*) such as photoplethysmography, heart rate, heart rate variability, respiratory rate, and oxygenation captured simultaneously. (*C*) Transcutaneous Piezoelectric Nanosensor for Cardiac Monitoring producing an ultrasonographic window to generate Doppler spectra analysis of systole and diastole time intervals, and tissue Doppler spectra synchronized with ECG.

INTEGRATION APPROACHES FOR WEARABLE AND DIGITAL HEALTH DEVICES WITHIN POPULATION HEALTH

While considering the integration of digital health technologies in the care armamentarium of patients with HF, it is crucial to take into account all key stakeholders, namely; patients and caregivers, physicians, and ambulatory clinic staff (especially the staff responsible for monitoring and acting on the incoming data), clinical practice administrative staff for operationalizing workflow and payors for billing and compliance policies.[2,71] From population health systems of care perspective, the use of a digital health technology should not only be supported by scientific data with evidence in favor of patient-reported metrics as well as clinical outcomes but also it should also address, and potentially overcome, important social determinants of health, access barriers, and be sensitive to patient needs across the population (see **Table 2**). Using our framework, we will review some of the needs and challenges of the key stakeholders.

Patients and Caregivers

Patients with HF typically represent an older cohort, with 2 to 3 medical co-illnesses. This represents a very distinct population from that of healthy adults using wearables such as an Apple watch for general health and fitness. Other barriers across a patient population include, varying health literacy and technology fluency, limited broadband access, privacy concerns, language barriers, and financial concerns.[1]

Physicians, Clinical Staff, and Health Care System Administration

For physicians considering digital health technologies for their patients with HF, the primary challenge often is finding the right platform or "one complete solution" given the broad risk spectrum of the patients with HF cohort. While most current digital health platforms offer the monitoring of biometric data, when it comes to data insights that are actionable or offer real-time risk-prediction, most of the current platforms/technologies are still in a nascent stage. Until machine learning models evolve further, the current signal-to-noise ratio is a major barrier for the implementation of digital health technologies, especially given the limited bandwidth of the clinical staff who must cater to many needs of patients including health education, addressing clinical concerns, prescription refills, and care coordination. In addition to the above, physicians are also reluctant to offer digital health technologies due to the fall-off in effective and sustained patient engagement over time. Multiple studies have shown that patient interest in any given digital health technology or wearable wanes with a dramatic fall-off 6-months postinitiation.[72] Many of the above reasons are also why health care administrative staff are reluctant to adopt digital health technologies which further thwarts adoption.

Billing and Compliance

Ultimately, for digital health technologies to play a larger role in health care delivery across a population, there should be aligned business incentives and financial reimbursement in a way similar to outpatient office visits. While monthly reimbursement for RPM is a step forward, it is still riddled with barriers and complexities both for patients as well as clinical practices with significant differences in compliance requirements and secondary copays. This issue is further compounded for patients using more than one digital health technology such as an patient with HF with diabetes or COPD using multiple digital health platforms.

THE FUTURE OF WEARABLE AND DIGITAL HEALTH TECHNOLOGIES IN HEART FAILURE

Undoubtedly, current digital health technologies facilitate the ability to interface with patient data in unprecedented and continuously evolving ways. In this review, we have introduced a novel characterization for the subtyping of HF digital phenotypes with progressively increasing digital granularity to construct a framework whereby clinicians and patients are able to extract maximum clinical utility offered by these digital devices. We have also outlined the various barriers that impede the application and integration of devices into clinical workflows. Only by systematically reviewing the evidence for existing digital health platforms are we able to contextualize the strengths and weaknesses of any given device, appropriately align datasets with the outcomes they should be measuring, and address the social determinants of health including patient engagement and digital health divides to finally provide actionable data and scalability in the treatment of patients with HF. As such, we foresee a successful translational implementation of digital health technologies in patients with HF by fully appreciating the digital phenotype that is constructed by any given device, creating standardized approaches to data collection, and applying scientific rigor and methodology to the evaluation of the efficacy of these devices in improving HF-related outcomes.

CLINICS CARE POINTS

- When considering a digital health device for any given patient, it is important to align the data being acquired against a practical and achievable outcome for that technology (eg, HF hospitalization, rather than mortality) and to further corroborate this data with patient-reported outcomes (PROs) such as quality of life measures.

- Mutual technology acceptance leverages the concept of patient "co-designs" and utilizes the following principles for implementation: (1) identifying the barriers for adoption at the individual level (2) testing the proposed adoption by assessing workflow enhancement and data accessibility to patients and caregivers (3) developing a pre and postimplementation strategy to enhance a patient's use of a new technology.

- Digital smartphone-based technologies that address long-term engagement include (1) text messaging to target medication adherence, (2) behavioral messaging that is disease-specific to promote lifestyle changes, (3) combining medication adherence with PROs of quality of life.

ICMJE STATEMENT OF AUTHORSHIP

Concept and design: All authors. Acquisition, analysis, and interpretation of data: All authors. Drafting of the manuscript: All authors. Critical revision of the manuscript for important intellectual content: All authors. Statistical analysis: N/A. Literature search: All authors. Obtained funding: S.P. Bhavnani. Administrative, technical, or material support: Bhavnani. Supervision: S.P. Bhavnani. Final approval of the version to be published: All authors.

ACKNOWLEDGMENTS

We wish to thank Xu Sheng PhD and Joe Wang PhD from the University of California San Diego, Maulik Majmudar MD MSc from Biofourmis, and Muthu Krishnan MBA from Kencor Health for their generous contribution of the figures as part of digital health phenotypes, and our appreciation to Alivecor, Abbott, Dexcom, and iHealthLabs for providing illustrations of digital health devices used within the examples of remote patient monitoring.

DISCLOSURES

RK: R. Khedraki, MD has no disclosures to report. AS: A.V. Srivastava MD is a clinical advisor to

AccurKardia and on the advisory board for Abiomed; receives speaking honoraria for Abbott and Medtronic. SB: S.P. Bhavnani MD is a scientific advisor to Analytics 4 Life and Blumio; consultant to Bristol Meyers Squibb, Pfizer, and Infineon; was a data safety monitoring board chair at Proteus Digital; has received research support from Scripps Clinic and the Qualcomm Foundation, and is member of the innovation advisory boards at the American College of Cardiology, American Society of Echocardiography, and BIO-COM (all non-profit institutions with all positions voluntary).

REFERENCES

1. Bhavnani SP, Narula J, Sengupta PP. Mobile technology and the digitization of healthcare. Eur Heart J 2016;37:1428–38.
2. Bhavnani SP, Parakh K, Atreja A, et al. 2017 Roadmap for Innovation-ACC health policy statement on healthcare transformation in the era of digital health, big data, and precision health: a report of the American College of Cardiology Task Force on Health Policy Statements and Systems of Care. J Am Coll Cardiol 2017;70:2696–718.
3. Bhatia A, Maddox TM. Remote patient monitoring in heart failure: factors for clinical efficacy. Int J Heart Fail 2021;3:31–50.
4. Bayoumy K, Gaber M, Elshafeey A, et al. Smart wearable devices in cardiovascular care: where we are and how to move forward. Nat Rev Cardiol 2021;18(8):581–99.
5. Setoguchi S, Stevenson LW, Schneeweiss S. Repeated hospitalizations predict mortality in the community population with heart failure. Am Heart J 2007;154:260–6.
6. Jackson SL, Tong X, King RJ, et al. National Burden of Heart Failure Events in the United States, 2006 to 2014. Circ Heart Fail 2018;11:e004873.
7. Jencks SF, Williams MV, Coleman EA. Rehospitalizations among patients in the Medicare fee-for-service program. N Engl J Med 2009;360:1418–28.
8. Greene SJ, Butler J, Albert NM, et al. Medical therapy for heart failure with reduced ejection fraction: the CHAMP-HF Registry. J Am Coll Cardiol 2018; 72:351–66.
9. Srivastava PK, DeVore AD, Hellkamp AS, et al. Heart failure hospitalization and guideline-directed prescribing patterns among heart failure with reduced ejection fraction patients. JACC Heart Fail 2021;9:28–38.
10. Maddox TM, Song Y, Allen J, et al. Trends in U.S. ambulatory cardiovascular care 2013 to 2017: JACC review topic of the week. J Am Coll Cardiol 2020;75:93–112.
11. Adamson PB. Pathophysiology of the transition from chronic compensated and acute decompensated heart failure: new insights from continuous monitoring devices. Curr Heart Fail Rep 2009;6:287–92.
12. Alvarez P, Sianis A, Brown J, et al. Chronic disease management in heart failure: focus on telemedicine and remote monitoring. Rev Cardiovasc Med 2021; 22:403–13.
13. Satici S, Iyngkaran P, Andrew S, et al. Rethinking heart failure care and health technologies from early COVID-19 experiences - A narrative review. Rev Cardiovasc Med 2021;22:105–14.
14. DeVore AD, Wosik J, Hernandez AF. The future of wearables in heart failure patients. JACC Heart Fail 2019;7:922–32.
15. Cartwright M, Hirani SP, Rixon L, et al. Effect of telehealth on quality of life and psychological outcomes over 12 months (Whole Systems Demonstrator telehealth questionnaire study): nested study of patient reported outcomes in a pragmatic, cluster randomised controlled trial. BMJ 2013;346:f653.
16. Koehler F, Koehler K, Deckwart O, et al. Efficacy of telemedical interventional management in patients with heart failure (TIM-HF2): a randomised, controlled, parallel-group, unmasked trial. Lancet 2018;392: 1047–57.
17. Koehler F, Winkler S, Schieber M, et al. Anker SD and telemedical interventional monitoring in heart failure I. Impact of remote telemedical management on mortality and hospitalizations in ambulatory patients with chronic heart failure: the telemedical interventional monitoring in heart failure study. Circulation 2011;123:1873–80.
18. Ong MK, Romano PS, Edgington S, et al. Fonarow GC and better effectiveness after transition-heart failure research G. Effectiveness of remote patient monitoring after discharge of hospitalized patients with heart failure: the better effectiveness after transition – heart failure (BEAT-HF) Randomized Clinical Trial. JAMA Intern Med 2016;176:310–8.
19. Kitsiou S, Vatani H, Pare G, et al. Effectiveness of mobile health technology interventions for patients with heart failure: systematic review and meta-analysis. Can J Cardiol 2021;37(8):1248–59.
20. Huckvale K, Venkatesh S, Christensen H. Toward clinical digital phenotyping: a timely opportunity to consider purpose, quality, and safety. NPJ Digit Med 2019;2:88.
21. Torous J, Kiang MV, Lorme J, et al. New tools for new research in psychiatry: a scalable and customizable platform to empower data driven smartphone research. JMIR Ment Health 2016;3:e16.
22. Onnela JP, Rauch SL. Harnessing smartphone-based digital phenotyping to enhance behavioral and mental health. Neuropsychopharmacology 2016;41:1691–6.
23. Venkatesh V, Bala H. Technology acceptance Model 3 and a research agenda on interventions. Decis Sci 2008;39:273–315.

24. Banbury A, Nancarrow S, Dart J, et al. Adding value to remote monitoring: co-design of a health literacy intervention for older people with chronic disease delivered by telehealth - the telehealth literacy project. Patient Educ Couns 2020;103:597–606.

25. Vangeepuram N, Mayer V, Fei K, et al. Smartphone ownership and perspectives on health apps among a vulnerable population in East Harlem, New York. Mhealth 2018;4:31.

26. Krishnaswami A, Beavers C, Dorsch MP, et al. Freeman AM, Bhavnani SP, Innovations CT and the geriatric cardiology councils ACoC. Gerotechnology for older adults with cardiovascular diseases: JACC State-of-the-Art Review. J Am Coll Cardiol 2020;76: 2650–70.

27. Khoja S, Durrani H, Scott RE, et al. Conceptual framework for development of comprehensive e-health evaluation tool. Telemed J E Health 2013; 19:48–53.

28. Bhavnani SP, Harzand A. From false-positives to technological Darwinism: controversies in digital health. Per Med 2018;15:247–50.

29. Pezel T, Berthelot E, Gauthier J, et al. Epidemiological characteristics and therapeutic management of patients with chronic heart failure who use smartphones: potential impact of a dedicated smartphone application (report from the OFICSel study). Arch Cardiovasc Dis 2021;114:51–8.

30. Bakogiannis C, Tsarouchas A, Mouselimis D, et al. A patient-oriented app (ThessHF) to improve self-care quality in heart failure: from evidence-based design to Pilot Study. JMIR Mhealth Uhealth 2021; 9:e24271.

31. Byambasuren O, Beller E, Glasziou P. Current knowledge and adoption of mobile health apps among australian general practitioners: Survey Study. JMIR Mhealth Uhealth 2019;7:e13199.

32. Lavallee DC, Lee JR, Austin E, et al. mHealth and patient generated health data: stakeholder perspectives on opportunities and barriers for transforming healthcare. Mhealth 2020;6:8.

33. Mortara A, Vaira L, Palmieri V, et al. Would you prescribe mobile health apps for heart failure self-care? An integrated review of commercially available mobile technology for heart failure patients. Card Fail Rev 2020;6:e13.

34. Agarwal S, LeFevre AE, Lee J, et al. Guidelines for reporting of health interventions using mobile phones: mobile health (mHealth) evidence reporting and assessment (mERA) checklist. BMJ 2016;352:i1174.

35. Cajita MI, Gleason KT, Han HR. A systematic review of mHealth-based heart failure interventions. J Cardiovasc Nurs 2016;31:E10–22.

36. Gabizon I, Bhagirath V, Lokker C, et al. What do physicians need to know in order to 'prescribe' mobile applications to patients with cardiovascular disease? Per Med 2019;16:263–8.

37. Bermon A, Uribe AF, Perez-Rivero PF, et al. Efficacy and safety of text messages targeting adherence to cardiovascular medications in secondary prevention: TXT2HEART colombia randomized controlled trial. JMIR Mhealth Uhealth 2021;9:e25548.

38. Glasgow RE, Knoepke CE, Magid D, et al. The NUDGE trial pragmatic trial to enhance cardiovascular medication adherence: study protocol for a randomized controlled trial. Trials 2021;22:528.

39. Schulz M, Griese-Mammen N, Schumacher PM, et al. The impact of pharmacist/physician care on quality of life in elderly heart failure patients: results of the PHARM-CHF randomized controlled trial. ESC Heart Fail 2020;7(6):3310–9.

40. Bhavnani SP. Digital health: opportunities and challenges to develop the next-generation technology-enabled models of cardiovascular care. Methodist Debakey Cardiovasc J 2020;16:296–303.

41. Omar M, Jensen J, Frederiksen PH, et al. Hemodynamic determinants of activity measured by accelerometer in patients with stable heart failure. JACC Heart Fail 2021;9:824–35.

42. Bui AL, Horwich TB, Fonarow GC. Epidemiology and risk profile of heart failure. Nat Rev Cardiol 2011;8: 30–41.

43. Cho JS, Shrestha S, Kagiyama N, et al. A network-based "phenomics" approach for discovering patient subtypes from high-throughput cardiac imaging data. JACC Cardiovasc Imaging 2020;13: 1655–70.

44. Shah SJ, Katz DH, Selvaraj S, et al. Phenomapping for novel classification of heart failure with preserved ejection fraction. Circulation 2015;131:269–79.

45. Majmudar MD, Dy Aungst T. Telemedicine in heart failure-ineffective or just ill used? JAMA Intern Med 2016;176:1035.

46. Farwati M, Riaz H, Tang WHW. Digital health applications in heart failure: a critical appraisal of literature. Curr Treat Options Cardiovasc Med 2021;23:12.

47. Marquis-Gravel G, Roe MT, Turakhia MP, et al. Technology-enabled clinical trials: transforming medical evidence generation. Circulation 2019;140:1426–36.

48. Kelkar AA, Spertus J, Pang P, et al. Utility of patient-reported outcome instruments in heart failure. JACC Heart Fail 2016;4:165–75.

49. Piotrowicz E, Pencina MJ, Opolski G, et al. Effects of a 9-Week hybrid comprehensive telerehabilitation program on long-term outcomes in patients with heart failure: the telerehabilitation in heart failure patients (TELEREH-HF) randomized clinical trial. JAMA Cardiol 2020;5:300–8.

50. Skov Schacksen C, Dyrvig AK, Henneberg NC, et al. Patient-reported outcomes from patients with heart failure participating in the future patient telerehabilitation program: data from the intervention arm of a randomized controlled trial. JMIR Cardio 2021;5: e26544.

51. Abraham WT, Adamson PB, Bourge RC, et al. Wireless pulmonary artery haemodynamic monitoring in chronic heart failure: a randomised controlled trial. Lancet 2011;377:658–66.

52. Heywood JT, Jermyn R, Shavelle D, et al. Impact of practice-based management of pulmonary artery pressures in 2000 patients implanted with the CardioMEMS sensor. Circulation 2017;135:1509–17.

53. Shavelle DM, Desai AS, Abraham WT, et al. Lower rates of heart failure and all-cause hospitalizations during pulmonary artery pressure-guided therapy for ambulatory heart failure: one-year outcomes from the CardioMEMS Post-Approval Study. Circ Heart Fail 2020;13:e006863.

54. Cowie MR, de Groote P, McKenzie S, et al. Rationale and design of the CardioMEMS Post-Market Multinational Clinical Study: COAST. ESC Heart Fail 2020;7: 865–72.

55. Desai AS, Bhimaraj A, Bharmi R, et al. Ambulatory hemodynamic monitoring reduces heart failure hospitalizations in "real-world" clinical practice. J Am Coll Cardiol 2017;69:2357–65.

56. Abraham J, Bharmi R, Jonsson O, et al. Association of ambulatory hemodynamic monitoring of heart failure with clinical outcomes in a concurrent matched cohort analysis. JAMA Cardiol 2019;4:556–63.

57. Benza RL, Doyle M, Lasorda D, et al. Monitoring pulmonary arterial hypertension using an implantable hemodynamic sensor. Chest 2019;156:1176–86.

58. Veenis JF, Radhoe SP, van Mieghem NM, et al. Safety and feasibility of hemodynamic pulmonary artery pressure monitoring using the CardioMEMS device in LVAD management. J Card Surg 2021;36:3271–80.

59. van Veldhuisen DJ, Braunschweig F, Conraads V, et al. Intrathoracic impedance monitoring, audible patient alerts, and outcome in patients with heart failure. Circulation 2011;124:1719–26.

60. Luthje L, Vollmann D, Seegers J, et al. A randomized study of remote monitoring and fluid monitoring for the management of patients with implanted cardiac arrhythmia devices. Europace 2015;17:1276–81.

61. Bohm M, Drexler H, Oswald H, et al. Fluid status telemedicine alerts for heart failure: a randomized controlled trial. Eur Heart J 2016;37:3154–63.

62. Maier SKG, Paule S, Jung W, et al. Evaluation of thoracic impedance trends for implant-based remote monitoring in heart failure patients - results from the (J-)HomeCARE-II Study. J Electrocardiol 2019;53:100–8.

63. Conraads VM, Tavazzi L, Santini M, et al. Sensitivity and positive predictive value of implantable intrathoracic impedance monitoring as a predictor of heart failure hospitalizations: the SENSE-HF trial. Eur Heart J 2011;32:2266–73.

64. Boehmer JP, Hariharan R, Devecchi FG, et al. A Multisensor Algorithm predicts heart failure events in patients with implanted devices: results from the MultiSENSE Study. JACC Heart Fail 2017;5:216–25.

65. Capucci A, Santini L, Favale S, et al. Preliminary experience with the multisensor HeartLogic algorithm for heart failure monitoring: a retrospective case series report. ESC Heart Fail 2019;6:308–18.

66. Santini L, D'Onofrio A, Dello Russo A, et al. Prospective evaluation of the multisensor HeartLogic algorithm for heart failure monitoring. Clin Cardiol 2020; 43:691–7.

67. Guk K, Han G, Lim J, et al. Evolution of wearable devices with real-time disease monitoring for personalized healthcare. Nanomaterials (Basel) 2019;9.

68. Un KC, Wong CK, Lau YM, et al. Observational study on wearable biosensors and machine learning-based remote monitoring of COVID-19 patients. Sci Rep 2021;11:4388.

69. Saner H, Schutz N, Botros A, et al. Potential of ambient sensor systems for early detection of health problems in older adults. Front Cardiovasc Med 2020;7:110.

70. Wang C, Qi B, Lin M, et al. Continuous monitoring of deep-tissue haemodynamics with stretchable ultrasonic phased arrays. Nat Biomed Eng 2021;5: 749–58.

71. Bhavnani SP, Sitapati AM. Virtual Care 2.0-a Vision for the future of data-driven technology-enabled healthcare. Curr Treat Options Cardiovasc Med 2019;21:21.

72. Meyerowitz-Katz G, Ravi S, Arnolda L, et al. Rates of attrition and dropout in app-based interventions for chronic disease: systematic review and meta-analysis. J Med Internet Res 2020;22:e20283.

73. Bakogiannis C, Tsarouchas A, Mouselimis D, et al. A patient-oriented app (ThessHF) to improve self-care quality in heart failure: from evidence-based design to pilot study. JMIR Mhealth Uhealth 2021; 9(4):e24271.

74. Dwinger S, Rezvani F, Kriston L, et al. Effects of telephone-based health coaching on patient-reported outcomes and health behavior change: a randomized controlled trial. PLoS One 2020;15(9): e0236861.

75. Pekmezaris R, Nouryan CN, Schwartz R, et al. A randomized controlled trial comparing telehealth self-management to standard outpatient management in underserved black and hispanic patients living with heart failure. Telemed J E Health 2019; 25(10):917–25.

76. Goldstein CM, Gathright EC, Dolansky MA, et al. Randomized controlled feasibility trial of two telemedicine medication reminder systems for older adults with heart failure. J Telemed Telecare 2014; 20(6):293–9.

77. Redfield MM, Anstrom KJ, Levine JA, et al. Isosorbide Mononitrate in Heart Failure with Preserved

Ejection Fraction. N Engl J Med 2015;373(24): 2314–24.

78. Koehler F, Winkler S, Schieber M, et al. Impact of remote telemedical management on mortality and hospitalizations in ambulatory patients with chronic heart failure: the telemedical interventional monitoring in heart failure study. Circulation 2011; 123(17):1873–80.

79. Ong MK, Romano PS, Edgington S, et al. Effectiveness of Remote Patient monitoring after discharge of hospitalized patients with heart failure: the better effectiveness after transition – heart failure (BEAT-HF) randomized clinical trial. JAMA Intern Med 2016;176(3):310–8.

80. Clays E, Puddu PE, Lustrek M, et al. Proof-of-concept trial results of the HeartMan mobile personal health system for self-management in congestive heart failure. Sci Rep 2021;11(1):5663.

81. Amir O, Ben-Gal T, Weinstein JM, et al. Evaluation of remote dielectric sensing (ReDS) technology-guided therapy for decreasing heart failure re-hospitalizations. Int J Cardiol 2017;240:279–84.

82. Lala A, Barghash MH, Giustino G, et al. Early use of remote dielectric sensing after hospitalization to reduce heart failure readmissions. ESC Heart Fail 2021;8(2):1047–54.

83. Inan OT, Baran Pouyan M, Javaid AQ, et al. Novel Wearable Seismocardiography and Machine Learning Algorithms Can Assess Clinical Status of Heart Failure Patients. Circ Heart Fail 2018;11(1): e004313.

84. Liu J, Yan B, Chen SC, et al. Non-Invasive Capillary Blood Pressure Measurement Enabling Early Detection and Classification of Venous Congestion. IEEE J Biomed Health Inform Aug 2021;25(8):2877–86.

85. Shah AJ, Isakadze N, Levantsevych O, et al. Detecting heart failure using wearables: a pilot study. Physiol Meas 2020;41(4):044001.

Machine Learning in Cardiovascular Imaging

Nobuyuki Kagiyama, MD, PhD[a,b], Márton Tokodi, MD, PhD[c], Partho P. Sengupta, MD, DM[d,*]

KEYWORDS

- Artificial intelligence • Machine learning • Deep learning • Cardiovascular imaging
- Echocardiography • Computed tomography • MRI

KEY POINTS

- The demand to improve the efficacy of the cardiovascular imaging workflow is growing continuously due to the increasing number of imaging study referrals.
- Machine learning can facilitate image acquisition and reconstruction, evaluate image quality, and automate the segmentation and interpretation of radiological images.
- Using raw image data or features extracted from radiological images, machine learning–based tools may also support diagnostic and therapeutic decisions, enhance precision phenotyping, and perform individualized risk stratification, ultimately leading to improved outcomes.
- Machine learning will be integrated into clinical practice, although there are still many challenges that we need to overcome.

INTRODUCTION

Artificial intelligence (AI) has become an integral part of our daily life; for example, we use face recognition to unlock smartphones, talk to smart speakers that analyze and execute our voice commands, and purchase products online recommended by AI algorithms. The core technology paradigm facilitating such advancements is machine learning (ML), a branch of AI that enables computers to learn sophisticated patterns and insights from the data without being explicitly programmed (**Fig. 1**). Currently, ML is attracting increased attention, which is attributable to 3 key factors: (1) the increasing ubiquity of large, multifaceted data sets; (2) the availability of relatively inexpensive and powerful computational resources; and (3) the advent of deep learning (DL) algorithms (ie, artificial neural networks having more than one hidden layer between the inputs and outputs). Over the past decade, a plethora of studies have been published exploring the

potential utility of ML in cardiovascular (CV) imaging, and some of the proposed tools have already been implemented in imaging applications. ML may improve several aspects of CV imaging, such as patient selection and referral, diagnostics, therapy planning, and prognostication.[1] Nevertheless, there are still many challenges that we need to overcome before these tools can be translated into clinical practice. In this review, we discuss the most promising applications of ML in CV imaging.

ML FOR IMAGING AUTOMATION AND INTERPRETATION

The amount and the complexity of imaging tests have been steadily increasing, and the number of readers is becoming insufficient.[2] As a result, time spent interpreting one image is getting shorter, the occurrence of misdiagnoses may increase, and half of the radiologists in the United States become a defendant by the age of 60

N. Kagiyama and M. Tokodi contributed equally to this work and are joint first authors.
[a] Department of Digital Health and Telemedicine R&D, Juntendo University, Tokyo, Japan; [b] Department of Cardiovascular Biology and Medicine, Juntendo University, Tokyo, Japan; [c] Heart and Vascular Center, Semmelweis University, Budapest, Hungary; [d] Division of Cardiovascular Diseases, Rutgers Robert Wood Johnson Medical School, 1 Robert Wood Johnson Place, New Brunswick, NJ 08901, USA
* Corresponding author.
E-mail address: partho.sengupta@rutgers.edu

Heart Failure Clin 18 (2022) 245–258
https://doi.org/10.1016/j.hfc.2021.11.003
1551-7136/22/

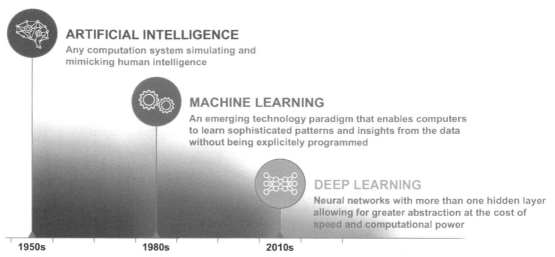

ARTIFICIAL INTELLIGENCE
Any computation system simulating and
mimicking human intelligence

MACHINE LEARNING
An emerging technology paradigm that enables computers
to learn sophisticated patterns and insights from the data
without being explicitly programmed

DEEP LEARNING
Neural networks with more than one hidden layer
allowing for greater abstraction at the cost of
speed and computational power

1950s   1980s   2010s

Fig. 1. Artificial intelligence, machine learning, and deep learning. *Artificial intelligence* is a broad and ambiguous term that describes any computational system mimicking human intelligence. *Machine learning*, traditionally considered a branch of artificial intelligence, is an emerging technology paradigm that enables computers to learn sophisticated patterns and insights from the data without being explicitly programmed. *Deep learning* is a subfield of machine learning that focuses on neural networks with more than one hidden layer.

years.[3] Accordingly, one of the essential tasks of ML in CV imaging is the automation of image interpretation. Although ML-based automated tools will significantly reduce the interpretation time and the incidence of misdiagnosis, it is yet unlikely that they will perform the entire image interpretation by themselves because of their limited capabilities and ethical and legal concerns. Nevertheless, regardless of the preference, it will be inevitable for clinicians to use these ML-based tools; thus, they should be familiar with the fundamental concepts of the underlying algorithms.

Image recognition, particularly image classification, is a common task in computer vision, which can also be applied to radiological image interpretation. Using a convolutional neural network (CNN)—a deep neural network aptly suited for image analysis—Madani and colleagues created a tool that automatically classified echocardiographic images into 15 echocardiographic views with high accuracy (**Fig. 2**A).[4] In addition to such view classification, Zhang and colleagues also trained a CNN to perform segmentation in echocardiographic images.[5] Their model depicted segments highly concordant with those drawn manually by CV imaging specialists, enabling the automated and accurate assessment of several functional and structural echocardiographic parameters (**Fig. 2**B).

Some of these automated view classification, segmentation, and measurement tools have begun to infiltrate our daily clinical practice. For example, when we measure global longitudinal strain, some of the latest echocardiography software solutions automatically identify 2-, 3-, and 4-chamber views from the acquired clips and trace the myocardium. Other applications can automatically recognize that the image is a pulse wave Doppler image at the left ventricular (LV) outflow tract and calculate stroke volume by automatically measuring the flow velocity curves. A couple of applications can even guide the acquisition of echocardiographic images. Caption Health and EchoNous have separately developed similar software solutions that evaluate the image quality and guide the operator in real-time to move the probe to improve the image (**Fig. 3**).[6] Both solutions are also capable of automatically quantifying the LV ejection fraction (LVEF). In cardiac magnetic resonance (CMR) imaging and computed tomography (CT), the latest applications automatically assist image acquisition with adjusting the region of interest and automatically segmenting anatomic structures.[7,8]

Most of these tools are enabled by training deep neural networks in a supervised manner. The reference to supervision indicates whether data have been labeled with the actual response or outcome (the ground truth), and algorithms that use labeled data are termed supervised learning techniques—a collection of ML algorithms attempting to model how independent variables relate to a dependent variable (ie, the label of interest). As opposed to supervised algorithms, unsupervised learning methods use unlabeled data, meaning there are no outcomes or prediction labels assigned to the data points. Thus, instead of fitting data to a

A

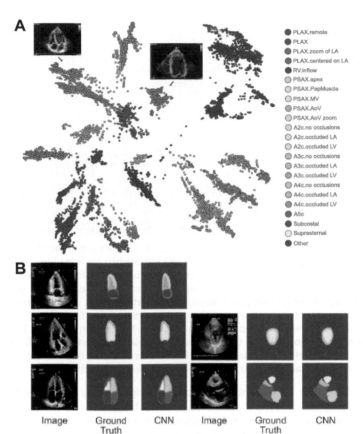

- ● PLAX.remote
- ● PLAX
- ● PLAX.zoom of LA
- ● PLAX.centered on LA
- ● RV.inflow
- ○ PSAX.apex
- ○ PSAX.PapMuscle
- ○ PSAX.MV
- ○ PSAX.AoV
- ○ PSAX.AoV zoom
- ○ A2c.no occlusions
- ○ A2c.occluded LA
- ○ A2c.occluded LV
- ○ A3c.no occlusions
- ○ A3c.occluded LA
- ○ A3c.occluded LV
- ○ A4c.no occlusions
- ○ A4c.occluded LA
- ○ A4c.occluded LV
- ● A5c
- ● Subcostal
- ○ Suprasternal
- ● Other

B

| Image | Ground Truth | CNN | Image | Ground Truth | CNN |

Fig. 2. Deep learning–based view classification and segmentation of echocardiographic images. (*A*) t-Distributed stochastic neighbor embedding was applied to visualize the results of the CNN-based view classification. The colors of dots correspond to different echocardiographic views. (*B*) Following view classification, another CNN model was used to segment cardiac chambers in 5 different echocardiographic views: A2c, A3c, A4c (left: top, middle, and bottom, respectively), PLAX at the level of the papillary muscle (right, middle), and PLAX (right, bottom). For each view, the trio of images, from left to right, corresponds to the original image, the manually traced image (ground truth), and the automatically segmented image. A2c, apical 2-chamber; A3c, apical 3-chamber; A4c, apical 4-chamber; A5c, apical 5-chamber; LA, left atrium; LV, left ventricle; PLAX, parasternal long axis. (*From* Zhang J, Gajjala S, Agrawal P, Tison GH, Hallock LA, Beussink-Nelson L, Lassen MH, Fan E, Aras MA, Jordan C, Fleischmann KE, Melisko M, Qasim A, Shah SJ, Bajcsy R, Deo RC. Fully Automated Echocardiogram Interpretation in Clinical Practice. Circulation. 2018 Oct 16;138(16):1623-1635.)

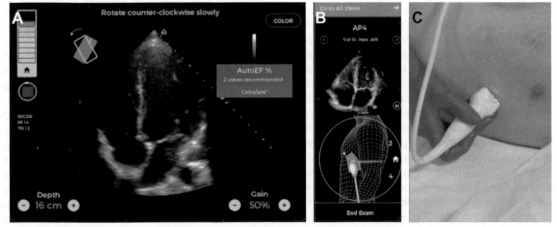

Fig. 3. Echocardiographic image acquisition guided by deep learning. The deep learning–based software guides the user to acquire diagnostic echocardiographic images (*A* and *B*) by appropriate positioning of the probe (*C*) and calculates left ventricular ejection fraction from the automatically acquired images. AP4, apical 4-chamber; EF, ejection fraction. (*From* Narang A, Bae R, Hong H, Thomas Y, Surette S, Cadieu C, Chaudhry A, Martin RP, McCarthy PM, Rubenson DS, Goldstein S, Little SH, Lang RM, Weissman NJ, Thomas JD. Utility of a Deep-Learning Algorithm to Guide Novices to Acquire Echocardiograms for Limited Diagnostic Use. JAMA Cardiol. 2021 Jun 1;6(6):624-632. Used with permission of Drs J. Thomas and Narang.)

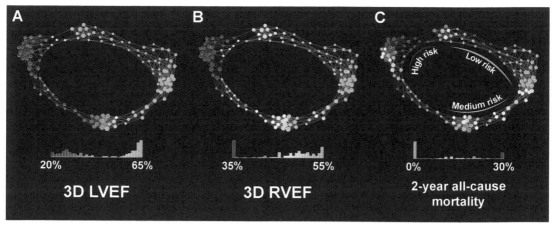

Fig. 4. Topological network of patients with cardiac disease (n = 174). The topological network was created using 7 echocardiographic features (3D left ventricular end-diastolic volume index, 3D left ventricular mass index, 3D left ventricular ejection fraction, 3D left ventricular longitudinal strain, 3D left ventricular circumferential strain, 3D right ventricular end-diastolic volume index, and 3D right ventricular ejection fraction) of heart failure patients with reduced left ventricular ejection fraction, heart transplant recipients and patients with severe primary mitral valve regurgitation. The generated network consists of nodes with edges between them. Each node represents a collection of similar patients, and 2 nodes are connected if they have at least 1 patient in common. Nodes are color-coded based on 3D left ventricular ejection fraction (*A*), 3D right ventricular ejection fraction (*B*), or 2-year all-cause mortality (*C*). Metric: normalized correlation, lenses: 2 × multidimensional scaling (resolution: 30, gain: 4.0, equalized). LVEF, left ventricular ejection fraction; RVEF, right ventricular ejection fraction.

prespecified result, these algorithms attempt to identify any potentially consistent, underlying patterns in the data. Typical applications of unsupervised algorithms include clustering analysis and dimensionality reduction.

PHENOTYPING AND RISK STRATIFICATION

Unsupervised learning may enable precision cardiology by synthesizing multiple domains of input features to subdivide monolithic disease categories (eg, heart failure [HF] or atrial fibrillation) into more stratified and personalized disease phenotypes that might respond differently to a given therapy. This idea is often termed precision phenotyping. Beyond the most frequently applied clustering algorithms (such as hierarchical or k-means clustering), there are other rapidly emerging approaches targeting the identification of novel, clinically relevant phenotypes. One such technique is topological data analysis (TDA), which adopts methods of topology, a discipline of mathematics focusing on shape analysis, to create compact visual representations of high-dimensional data sets (**Fig. 4**).[9] TDA amalgamates unsupervised pattern detection and network visualization by identifying and connecting data points (ie, patients) with very similar characteristics in a multidimensional space and then plotting the data as a topological network in a lower-dimensional space. The generated network consists of nodes (representing collections of similar patients) connected by edges if they have at least 1 patient in common. These networks can be color-coded based on the outcome of interest to reveal clinically meaningful regions (ie, phenotypes). TDA and other clustering algorithms have been widely applied on CV imaging data to uncover distinct phenotypes of aortic stenosis severity,[10] to identify novel phenogroups in HF patients with preserved EF (HFpEF),[11,12] or to explore the entire spectrum of cardiac function, from normal to end-stage HF.[13,14] Of note, the identification of novel phenotypes often represents only the first step in data analysis pipelines: the identified phenotypes can be used to label patients; then, the newly labeled data can be exploited by a subsequent supervised learning step to train models for risk stratification.[15]

In addition to improving the phenotyping of CV diseases, ML techniques can be leveraged to accurately predict different outcomes such as rehospitalization,[13] mortality,[16,17] or response to specific therapies.[15,18] The personalized prediction of outcomes is fundamental to patient-centered care, optimizing treatment strategies, and informing patients as part of shared decision-making.

ML IN SPECIFIC AREAS OF CV IMAGING

If designed, validated, and implemented appropriately, ML-based tools hold promises to revolutionize CV research and clinical care leading to an optimized day-to-day clinical workflow with improved diagnostics, risk assessment, and ultimately outcomes. In this section, we showcase the potentials of ML in various cherry-picked clinical scenarios that CV imaging professionals encounter in everyday clinical practice.

CT Analysis in Coronary Artery Disease

CT, mainly coronary CT angiography (CCTA), has gained pivotal importance in diagnosing and monitoring coronary artery disease (CAD). Consequently, the number of cardiac CT studies has been steadily growing, leading to an ever-increasing workload of CV imaging professionals.[19] ML may offer a way to aid clinicians in tackling this challenge as it can automate and improve various steps of CT analysis.

Identifying anatomically significant stenotic lesions in CCTA is a crucial but challenging task with substantial interobserver variability, which might be reduced using ML-based automated approaches.[20] First, ML can be deployed to guide and verify coronary artery centerline extraction.[21] Then, the extracted centerlines can be used to reconstruct CCTA volumes into images that enable better plaque visualization and identification. Several research groups have used features derived from cross-sectional images along the coronary artery centerline in ML models to determine whether the image contains a noncalcified plaque,[22,23] whereas others used such features to classify lesion segments as either healthy or diseased.[24] Moreover, several ML models have been implemented to automatically determine the degree of coronary stenosis using CCTA scans.[25-27] Importantly, the identification of plaques or stenoses is often only a prerequisite for prognostication, and CCTA-derived measures of coronary stenosis can be integrated into ML models to improve prognostication.[17]

The functional significance of a lesion, which might be even more important than its anatomic significance, can also be assessed with the assistance of ML techniques (**Fig. 5**). Itu and colleagues proposed an artificial neural network model to predict a fractional flow reserve value for each segment in the coronary artery tree.[28] Although its diagnostic and incremental prognostic value was demonstrated thoroughly,[29-31] this approach relies heavily on the geometry of the coronary artery tree model and is hence susceptible to the errors of the segmentation process. Therefore, other methods that skip coronary artery centerline extraction and lumen segmentation have also been proposed.[32]

In addition to the presence and significance of stenotic lesions, the extent of coronary artery calcification—expressed using the Agatston score—is also an independent and robust predictor of adverse CV events.[33] In current clinical practice, coronary artery calcium (CAC) scoring from ECG-gated non–contrast-enhanced cardiac CT scans requires manual actions performed by a human operator. ML could automate and accelerate this process, as several studies applying such algorithms have yielded promising results in predicting CAC scores and flagging ambiguous cases for expert review.[34-37] Moreover, with the help of ML-based tools, CAC scores can also be derived from chest CT examinations performed due to noncardiac indications, such as lung cancer screening or radiation therapy planning.[38-40]

Noncontrast cardiac CT scans can also be used to assess epicardial adipose tissue, which modulates coronary arterial function and is associated with adverse cardiac events.[41] To automate the quantification of epicardial adipose tissue, Commandeur and colleagues developed a CNN-based method, which exhibited a robust correlation with expert manual measurements.[42] In a subsequent study, they used this tool for the prognostication of asymptomatic subjects without known CAD. The ML-derived epicardial adipose tissue volume was found to be independently associated with an increased risk of major adverse cardiac events.[43] These findings imply that the ML-enabled rapid and automated assessment of epicardial adipose tissue has the potential to be incorporated into the routine reporting of noncontrast cardiac CT scans, providing incremental information on CV risk.

CMR Imaging in Cardiomyopathies

Cardiomyopathies represent a heterogeneous group of cardiac disorders characterized by structural and functional abnormalities of the myocardium, which cannot be explained by loading conditions or CAD.[44] CMR imaging plays a pivotal role in this patient population as it can provide valuable insights into the underlying etiology through the extensive characterization of the myocardium using techniques such as late gadolinium enhancement (LGE), T1 and T2 mapping.[45] Nonetheless, manual analysis is time-consuming and is prone to interobserver variability; thus, the ML-enabled automation of CMR image analysis would be desirable. Motivated by this, Augusto and colleagues have implemented a CNN-based tool to automate the segmentation of the left ventricle and the measurement of LV maximum wall thickness in noncontrast cine CMR images of patients with hypertrophic cardiomyopathy

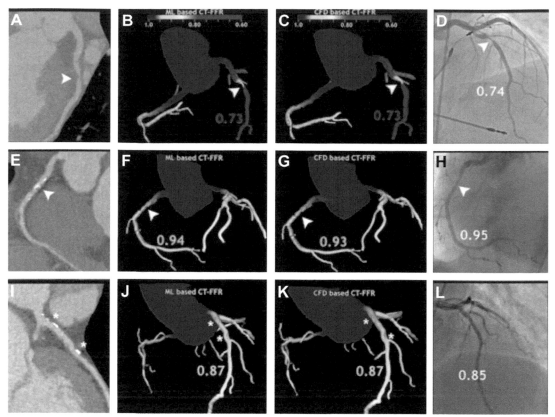

Fig. 5. A machine learning approach to assess coronary computed tomographic angiography–based fractional flow reserve. Two patients both with moderate (>50%) stenosis (*arrowheads*) and 1 patient with 2 serial mild stenoses (25%–49% indicated with an *asterisk* [*]) on CT angiography (*A, E, I*). In the first patient (*A–D*), machine learning ML-based CT-FFR predicts functionally obstructive stenosis in the mid-LAD with an ML-based CT-FFR value of 0.73 (*B*). CFD-based CT-FFR provided an identical result with a CT-FFR value of 0.73. Invasive angiography confirmed functionally obstructive stenosis with an invasive FFR of 0.74 (*D*). In the second patient (*E–H*), ML-based CT-FFR predicts the stenosis in the proximal right coronary artery as nonsignificant with an ML-based CT-FFR value of 0.94 (*E*). Invasive angiography (*H*) shows the stenosis. However, invasive FFR confirmed nonfunctionally obstructive stenosis with an invasive FFR of 0.95. In the third patient (*I–L*), the 2 serial mild stenoses in the LAD are predicted as nonsignificant with both ML-based and CFD-based CT-FFR. Invasive FFR confirmed the nonfunctionally of the lesions with an invasive FFR of 0.85. CFD, computational fluid dynamics; FFR, fractional flow reserve; LAD, left anterior descending artery. (*From* Coenen A, Kim YH, Kruk M, Tesche C, De Geer J, Kurata A, Lubbers ML, Daemen J, Itu L, Rapaka S, Sharma P, Schwemmer C, Persson A, Schoepf UJ, Kepka C, Hyun Yang D, Nieman K. Diagnostic Accuracy of a Machine-Learning Approach to Coronary Computed Tomographic Angiography-Based Fractional Flow Reserve: Result From the MACHINE Consortium. Circ Cardiovasc Imaging. 2018 Jun;11(6):e007217.)

(HCM).[46] In this study, their model yielded a precision superior to human experts with potential implications for diagnosis, risk stratification, and clinical trials (**Fig. 6**). Another group of researchers used a CNN-based method to enable the fast, automated, and accurate quantification of LGE myocardial scar volume, which is an important prognostic marker in patients with HCM.[47] Although these 2 studies focused on particular tasks, others sought to implement a more complex DL-based framework to perform entirely automated cardiac analysis from cine CMR images. An excellent example of this concept was

provided by Ruijsink and colleagues, who designed and validated a DL-based pipeline for the automated, quality-controlled segmentation and measurements of multiple left and right ventricular (RV) parameters using cine CMR images.[48]

To aid clinicians in accurately identifying the underlying etiology of LV hypertrophy, ML can also be coupled with the texture analysis of CMR images. This was exemplified by Neisius and colleagues, whose support vector machine-based model using texture features (extracted from native T1 maps) achieved an area under the receiver-operating characteristic curve of 0.89 in

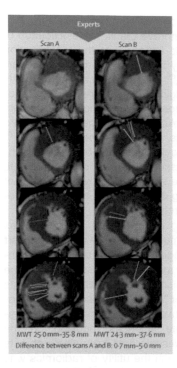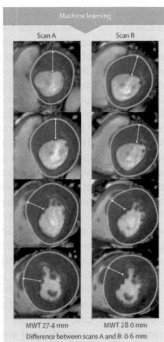

MWT 25·0 mm–35·8 mm MWT 24·3 mm–37·6 mm
Difference between scans A and B: 0·7 mm–5·0 mm

MWT 27·4 mm MWT 28·0 mm
Difference between scans A and B: 0·6 mm

Fig. 6. Machine learning–based cardiac MRI analysis to quantify left ventricular wall thickness in patients with hypertrophic cardiomyopathy. Within the same scan, experts picked different segments and locations in the myocardium and even different slices to measure MWT, leading to considerable disagreement in MWT measurement. Between tests, some experts changed their measurements to a completely different location or slice, leading to remarkable test-retest differences. On the other hand, the deep learning–based model showed higher intertest concordance than the human experts. MWT, maximum wall thickness. (*From* Augusto JB, Davies RH, Bhuva AN, Knott KD, Seraphim A, Alfarih M, Lau C, Hughes RK, Lopes LR, Shiwani H, Treibel TA, Gerber BL, Hamilton-Craig C, Ntusi NAB, Pontone G, Desai MY, Greenwood JP, Swoboda PP, Captur G, Cavalcante J, Bucciarelli-Ducci C, Petersen SE, Schelbert E, Manisty C, Moon JC. Diagnosis and risk stratification in hypertrophic cardiomyopathy using machine learning wall thickness measurement: a comparison with human test-retest performance. Lancet Digit Health. 2021 Jan;3(1):e20-e28. Reprinted with permission from Elsevier.)

distinguishing between HCM and hypertensive heart disease.[49] Moreover, as demonstrated by Satriano and colleagues, ML can also be used to accurately distinguish HCM from cardiac amyloidosis, Anderson-Fabry disease, and hypertensive cardiomyopathy using data from 3D myocardial deformation analysis of cine CMR images.[50]

Beyond the diagnosis of HCM, ML can also facilitate the detection of HCM mutations through the analysis of nonenhanced CMR cine images,[51] and the identification of HCM patients with ventricular tachyarrhythmia through texture analysis of LGE-positive areas.[52]

Notably, the application of ML is not limited to HCM, as it has been successfully applied to objectively diagnose dilated cardiomyopathy (DCM) using texture features extracted from T1 maps,[53] to predict response to medical therapy in patients with idiopathic DCM using CMR imaging–derived regional strain parameters,[54] or to risk-stratify patients with severe DCM or LV noncompaction cardiomyopathy.[55,56]

Echocardiography in HF

Echocardiography has been the cornerstone of HF characterization and management for decades. Nevertheless, the interpretation of echocardiograms requires a skilled reader, and measurements are subject to inter-reader variability. ML algorithms can be used to perform an automated and objective evaluation of echocardiograms to mitigate the effect of this factor. To this end, Zhang and colleagues implemented a CNN capable of identifying echocardiographic views with high accuracy and calculating LVEF and longitudinal strain when compared with manual tracings, respectively, as mentioned earlier.[5] Ouyang and colleagues reported another exciting approach: they trained a 3D CNN on full-length echocardiographic videos containing more cardiac cycles instead of manually selected still images at end-systole and end-diastole.[57] Their model could predict LVEF with a mean absolute error of 4.1% and 6.0% (compared with manual tracings) and reliably identified HF patients with reduced EF in internal and external test sets. Although the 2 methods mentioned earlier have notable differences, both rely on image segmentation. In contrast, Asch and colleagues proposed a DL-based model, which estimates EF directly from still echocardiographic images without performing image segmentation and volume measurements.[58] Their model achieved an accuracy of 0.92 for the detection LVEF ≤ 35%. Of note, instead of raw image data, standard echocardiographic parameters or velocity, strain, and strain rate traces can also be used to train ML algorithms to diagnose HF.[59–61]

Risk stratification is another crucial task in HF, and there is an increasing body of evidence that

ML can augment it. Significant strides have been achieved with ML models trained using the combination of echocardiographic measurements and other clinical variables.[62–65] Notably, these studies used hand-crafted echocardiographic parameters instead of analyzing the raw image data. Although human-derived metrics have well-established prognostic value and are easily interpretable, an approach not hindered by the limitations of human perception and pattern-recognition ability may further improve the predictive performance. Inspired by this idea, Ulloa-Cerna and colleagues trained a deep neural network using raw echocardiographic videos of an unselected patient cohort to predict 1-year all-cause mortality.[66] When tested in an independent data set of 2404 HF patients, their model exhibited superior performance than the Seattle Heart Failure score (area under the receiver-operating characteristic curve: 0.76 vs 0.70).

Instead of predicting outcomes directly, ML can be used to classify patients into newly identified phenotypes associated with different rates of adverse events. Recently, our research group has demonstrated the feasibility of this concept through 2 subsequent studies. First, we used TDA to integrate LV structural and functional echocardiographic features into a patient-patient similarity network in which we identified low-risk and high-risk regions (ie, phenotypes).[13] Then, we assigned each patient a label based on their location in the topological network, and we trained a deep neural network to classify them.[15] When we tested our model externally in HFpEF cohorts, patients classified as belonging to the high-risk phenotype showed higher rates of HF hospitalization or cardiac death than those classified as having low-risk.

EMERGING ML-BASED TECHNIQUES FOR THE ANALYSIS OF RADIOLOGICAL IMAGES

The field of ML is continuously evolving, and several new ML-based image analysis techniques have emerged over the past years. In this section, we will briefly discuss 2 of these: (1) generative adversarial networks (GANs) and (2) radiomics.

GANs are algorithmic architectures consisting of 2 deep neural networks pitted against each other to generate synthetic (ie, fake) images that resemble real ones. One of the neural networks (the generator) creates de novo images, whereas the other one (the discriminator) decides whether each image belongs to the actual training set or is it a synthetic one. As demonstrated by Zhang and colleagues, GANs can be implemented to generate LGE images from native T1 mapping images without contrast administration (**Fig. 7**).[67] GANs can also improve the view classification of echocardiographic images and the identification of LV hypertrophy in apical 4-chamber echocardiogram images.[68] Other applications of GAN models to CV imaging include increasing the resolution of CMR images,[69] or creating large amounts of realistically looking CMR images even in rare cardiac conditions, such as Tetralogy of Fallot.[70] The latter is an excellent example of data augmentation, which is essential to train data-hungry DL algorithms in case we cannot provide a sufficient amount of training data (which is a common scenario in CV research).

By representing pictorial data using complex mathematical formulae, radiomics aims to convert radiological images into structured, high-dimensional, and mineable data sets that can be supplied to ML algorithms. Its name refers to its similarities to other "omics" approaches (eg, genomics, transcriptomics, proteomics) that are specific fields of life sciences focusing on the generation of largescale data from single objects or samples. Although the utility of radiomics was first demonstrated in oncology,[71] CV imaging is another clinical discipline that could significantly benefit from the utilization of this emerging technology. Radiomics can be performed on standard-of-care images acquired using various imaging modalities. In echocardiography, our research group demonstrated that both myocardial function and fibrosis could be assessed from static images using radiomics (**Fig. 8**).[72] There has also been an increasing interest in the application of radiomics analysis to cardiac CT images, as it has achieved promising results in the characterization of coronary plaques and perivascular fat.[73,74] Moreover, proof-of-concept studies have demonstrated the feasibility and clinical value of CMR imaging–based radiomics in the diagnosis of HCM and the assessment of myocardial viability.[75,76] Thus, these studies imply that radiomics has the potential to become a useful tool in the clinical arena and will permanently transform CV imaging.

CONCERNS AND BARRIERS TO CLINICAL APPLICATION OF ML

As discussed so far, several studies have demonstrated the potentials of ML in CV imaging, and there are more and more commercially available applications. However, the vast majority of models reported in such studies have not been implemented in clinical practice. One of the most significant barriers in the application of research-reported models is the lack of generalizability. As ML

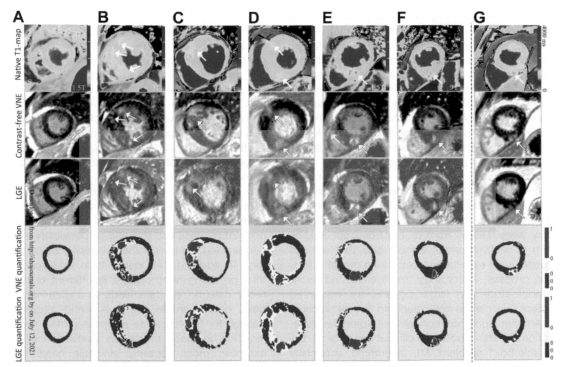

Fig. 7. Generative adversarial network-enabled virtual native enhancement for gadolinium-free cardiovascular magnetic resonance tissue characterization in hypertrophic cardiomyopathy. Examples to illustrate visuospatial agreement between GAN-enabled VNE and conventional LGE. T1 colormaps (top row) were adjusted individually to highlight the T1 signals corresponding to VNE signals. The bottom 2 rows visualize lesion regions by VNE and LGE using progressive thresholding (full width at half, a quarter, and eighth maximum) displayed with different colors. (A–F) A high visuospatial agreement was observed between VNE and LGE. Yellow arrows point to slightly different right ventricle sizes in VNE and LGE, suggesting patient movement between acquisitions. (G) An example of VNE displaying subtle changes more clearly than LGE. VNE, virtual native enhancement. (*From* Zhang Q, Burrage MK, Lukaschuk E, Shanmuganathan M, Popescu IA, Nikolaidou C, Mills R, Werys K, Hann E, Barutcu A, Polat SD; Hypertrophic Cardiomyopathy Registry (HCMR) Investigators, Salerno M, Jerosch-Herold M, Kwong RY, Watkins HC, Kramer CM, Neubauer S, Ferreira VM, Piechnik SK. Toward Replacing Late Gadolinium Enhancement With Artificial Intelligence Virtual Native Enhancement for Gadolinium-Free Cardiovascular Magnetic Resonance Tissue Characterization in Hypertrophic Cardiomyopathy. Circulation. 2021 Aug 24;144(8):589-599.)

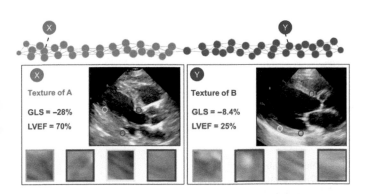

Fig. 8. Radiomics analysis of myocardial texture in echocardiographic images. Using myocardial texture features extracted from still echocardiographic images (*colored boxes*), an ML model was capable of identifying high-risk myocardium with reduced systolic function. In this figure, two representative examples are provided: patient X with normal systolic function and patient Y, who had significantly impaired systolic function. GLS, global longitudinal strain; LVEF, left ventricular ejection fraction. (*From* Kagiyama N, Shrestha S, Cho JS, Khalil M, Singh Y, Challa A, Casaclang-Verzosa G, Sengupta PP. A low-cost texture-based pipeline for predicting myocardial tissue remodeling and fibrosis using cardiac ultrasound. EBioMedicine. 2020 Apr;54:102726.)

algorithms are so complex that they can efficiently learn very fine details, they often capture unique characteristics of a given data set too specifically. This phenomenon is often referred to as overfitting. For example, if a model is trained using data from a particular hospital where all patients with HF undergo echocardiography using the same echo machine, the model may learn the characteristics of the images of that echo machine as a marker of high-risk patients. This model will perform poorly in other hospitals (ie, external data sets) as it learned clinically irrelevant details of the image instead of relevant associations between the images and patients' risk. Most of the published models suffer from the lack of generalizability as they were derived from proof-of-concept studies with a relatively small sample size that did not involve such external test sets in the model validation process. Accordingly, multicenter and multivendor studies in larger cohorts are warranted before they can be integrated into clinical practice.

Another significant concern regarding the application of ML models in clinical practice is the "black box" problem. ML algorithms, especially DL algorithms, are too complex, and even ML experts cannot usually explain why the model made a particular decision. However, when making life-changing decisions on diagnosis or treatment, it

would be pivotal to know the reasons behind them. In addition, when physicians face an ML prediction being different from their intuition, it will be challenging to decide whether they should rely on the model or their intuition. To overcome the problem of explainability, explainable AI is now one of the most intensively investigated topics in ML. However, research is still ongoing, and the "black box" problem remains a concern.

Ethical and legal issues represent another challenge for the application of ML in CV medicine. Transparency, justice, fairness, nonmaleficence, and responsibility are often discussed as ethical viewpoints.[77,78] As the ML model itself is often nonexplainable, transparency of the model development process and defining responsibility of the decision (eg, the user or the developer) are mandatory. In addition, ML learns from existing data; thus, providing inappropriate, insufficient, or incorrectly categorized data leads to a data set that does not resemble the real world accurately enough for ML to create a representative model, resulting in poor prediction performance. For example, most currently available health care data are collected in developed countries; therefore, ML models may be more suitable for such countries and make wrong decisions on socially vulnerable people. Also, regulatory frameworks

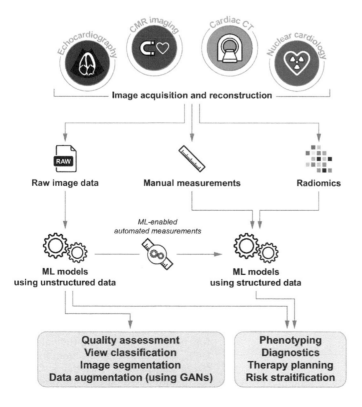

Fig. 9. The potential applications of machine learning in cardiovascular imaging.

have not been standardized as AI and ML are evolving rapidly. Legal challenges, including safety and effectiveness, liability, data protection, privacy, cybersecurity, and intellectual property law, are also yet to be addressed.[79] Researchers, clinicians, patients, manufacturers, and regulatory authorities must work together on tackling these challenges to ensure that ML benefits the entire society.

SUMMARY

ML represents an emerging technology paradigm with the potential to improve and accelerate the CV imaging workflow (**Fig. 9**). At image acquisition, ML will guide how to move the transducer and optimize the radiation dose of CT. Then, the acquired images can be analyzed using ML-based image recognition and segmentation tools. In addition, ML may even support diagnostic and therapeutic decisions. Nevertheless, the lack of generalizability and explainability remains a significant challenge. If current efforts are able to circumvent these barriers, ML will become a valuable tool in the clinical arena and will revolutionize CV imaging. Eventually, the emergence of AI techniques will allow physicians to create digital twins based on radiological images to explore the impact of therapeutic interventions and to aid personalized decision-making.

CLINICS CARE POINTS

- Machin learning is emerging as one of the most important evolutions in cardiovascular imaging, providing better imaging workflow and additional values extracting more information from images.
- Consider ethical and legal issues when implementing a machine learning model into your clinical practice.

DISCLOSURE

Dr N. Kagiyama is affiliated with a department funded by Philips Healthcare; Asahi KASEI Corporation; Inter Reha Co., Ltd.; and Toho Holdings Co., Ltd. based on collaborative research agreements, and receives research grant from EchoNous Inc. Dr M. Tokodi was supported by the New National Excellence Program (ÚNKP-20-3-II-SE-54) of the Ministry for Innovation and Technology in Hungary; the National Research, Development and Innovation Fund of Hungary (NKFIA; NVKP_16-1-2016-0017 - National Heart Program); and the Thematic Excellence Program (2020-4.1.1.-TKP2020) of the Ministry for Innovation and Technology in Hungary, within the framework of the Therapeutic Development and Bioimaging programs of the Semmelweis University. Dr P.P. Sengupta is a consultant for Ultromics, RCE Technologies, and Kencor Health.

REFERENCES

1. Sermesant M, Delingette H, Cochet H, et al. Applications of artificial intelligence in cardiovascular imaging. Nat Rev Cardiol 2021;18(8):600–9.
2. Papolos A, Narula J, Bavishi C, et al. Hospital use of echocardiography: insights from the nationwide inpatient sample. J Am Coll Cardiol 2016;67(5):502–11.
3. Baker SR, Whang JS, Luk L, et al. The demography of medical malpractice suits against radiologists. Radiology 2013;266(2):539–47.
4. Madani A, Arnaout R, Mofrad M, et al. Fast and accurate view classification of echocardiograms using deep learning. NPJ Digit Med 2018;1. https://doi.org/10.1038/s41746-017-0013-1.
5. Zhang J, Gajjala S, Agrawal P, et al. Fully Automated Echocardiogram Interpretation in Clinical Practice. Circulation 2018;138(16):1623–35.
6. Narang A, Bae R, Hong H, et al. Utility of a deep-learning algorithm to guide novices to acquire echocardiograms for limited diagnostic use. JAMA Cardiol 2021;6(6):624–32.
7. Bai W, Sinclair M, Tarroni G, et al. Automated cardiovascular magnetic resonance image analysis with fully convolutional networks. J Cardiovasc Magn Reson 2018;20(1):65.
8. Lell MM, Kachelrieß M. Recent and upcoming technological developments in computed tomography: high speed, low dose, deep learning, multienergy. Invest Radiol 2020;55(1):8–19.
9. Lum PY, Singh G, Lehman A, et al. Extracting insights from the shape of complex data using topology. Sci Rep 2013;3(1):1236.
10. Casaclang-Verzosa G, Shrestha S, Khalil MJ, et al. Network tomography for understanding phenotypic presentations in aortic stenosis. JACC Cardiovasc Imaging 2019;12(2):236–48.
11. Hedman Å K, Hage C, Sharma A, et al. Identification of novel pheno-groups in heart failure with preserved ejection fraction using machine learning. Heart 2020;106(5):342–9.
12. Przewlocka-Kosmala M, Marwick TH, Dabrowski A, et al. Contribution of Cardiovascular Reserve to Prognostic Categories of Heart Failure With Preserved Ejection Fraction: A Classification Based on Machine Learning. J Am Soc Echocardiogr 2019;32(5):604–15.e6.

13. Tokodi M, Shrestha S, Bianco C, et al. Interpatient similarities in cardiac function: a platform for personalized cardiovascular medicine. JACC Cardiovasc Imaging 2020;13(5):1119–32.

14. Cho JS, Shrestha S, Kagiyama N, et al. A network-based "phenomics" approach for discovering patient subtypes from high-throughput cardiac imaging data. JACC Cardiovasc Imaging 2020;13(8):1655–70.

15. Pandey A, Kagiyama N, Yanamala N, et al. Deep-learning models for the echocardiographic assessment of diastolic dysfunction. JACC Cardiovasc Imaging 2021. https://doi.org/10.1016/j.jcmg.2021.04.010.

16. Bello GA, Dawes TJW, Duan J, et al. Deep learning cardiac motion analysis for human survival prediction. Nat Mach Intell 2019;1:95–104.

17. Motwani M, Dey D, Berman DS, et al. Machine learning for prediction of all-cause mortality in patients with suspected coronary artery disease: a 5-year multicentre prospective registry analysis. Eur Heart J 2017;38(7):500–7.

18. Cikes M, Sanchez-Martinez S, Claggett B, et al. Machine learning-based phenogrouping in heart failure to identify responders to cardiac resynchronization therapy. Eur J Heart Fail 2019;21(1):74–85.

19. Levin DC, Parker L, Halpern EJ, et al. Coronary CT angiography: reversal of earlier utilization trends. J Am Coll Radiol 2019,16(2):147–55.

20. Arbab-Zadeh A, Hoe J. Quantification of coronary arterial stenoses by multidetector CT angiography in comparison with conventional angiography methods, caveats, and implications. JACC Cardiovasc Imaging 2011;4(2):191–202.

21. Wolterink JM, van Hamersvelt RW, Viergever MA, et al. Coronary artery centerline extraction in cardiac CT angiography using a CNN-based orientation classifier. Med Image Anal 2019;51:46–60.

22. Jawaid MM, Riaz A, Rajani R, et al. Framework for detection and localization of coronary non-calcified plaques in cardiac CTA using mean radial profiles. Comput Biol Med 2017;89:84–95.

23. Wei J, Zhou C, Chan HP, et al. Computerized detection of noncalcified plaques in coronary CT angiography: evaluation of topological soft gradient prescreening method and luminal analysis. Med Phys 2014;41(8):081901.

24. Zuluaga MA, Hush D, Delgado Leyton EJ, et al. Learning from only positive and unlabeled data to detect lesions in vascular CT images. Med Image Comput Comput Assist Interv 2011;14(Pt 3):9–16.

25. Kang D, Dey D, Slomka PJ, et al. Structured learning algorithm for detection of nonobstructive and obstructive coronary plaque lesions from computed tomography angiography. J Med Imaging (Bellingham) 2015;2(1):014003.

26. Kelm BM, Mittal S, Zheng Y, et al. Detection, grading and classification of coronary stenoses in computed tomography angiography. Med Image Comput Comput Assist Interv 2011;14(Pt 3):25–32.

27. Hong Y, Commandeur F, Cadet S, et al. Deep learning-based stenosis quantification from coronary CT Angiography. Proc SPIE Int Soc Opt Eng 2019;10949. https://doi.org/10.1117/12.2512168.

28. Itu L, Rapaka S, Passerini T, et al. A machine-learning approach for computation of fractional flow reserve from coronary computed tomography. J Appl Physiol (1985) 2016;121(1):42–52.

29. Yu M, Lu Z, Li W, et al. CT morphological index provides incremental value to machine learning based CT-FFR for predicting hemodynamically significant coronary stenosis. Int J Cardiol 2018;265:256–61.

30. Coenen A, Kim YH, Kruk M, et al. Diagnostic accuracy of a machine-learning approach to coronary computed tomographic angiography-based fractional flow reserve: result from the MACHINE Consortium. Circ Cardiovasc Imaging 2018;11(6):e007217.

31. Baumann S, Renker M, Schoepf UJ, et al. Gender differences in the diagnostic performance of machine learning coronary CT angiography-derived fractional flow reserve -results from the MACHINE registry. Eur J Radiol 2019;119:108657.

32. Kumamaru KK, Fujimoto S, Otsuka Y, et al. Diagnostic accuracy of 3D deep-learning-based fully automated estimation of patient-level minimum fractional flow reserve from coronary computed tomography angiography. Eur Heart J Cardiovasc Imaging 2020;21(4):437–45.

33. Budoff MJ, Shaw LJ, Liu ST, et al. Long-term prognosis associated with coronary calcification: observations from a registry of 25,253 patients. J Am Coll Cardiol 2007;49(18):1860–70.

34. van Velzen SGM, Lessmann N, Velthuis BK, et al. Deep learning for automatic calcium scoring in CT: validation using multiple cardiac CT and chest CT protocols. Radiology 2020;295(1):66–79.

35. Wolterink JM, Leiner T, Takx RA, et al. Automatic coronary calcium scoring in non-contrast-enhanced ECG-Triggered Cardiac CT with ambiguity detection. IEEE Trans Med Imaging 2015;34(9):1867–78.

36. Wolterink JM, Leiner T, de Vos BD, et al. Automatic coronary artery calcium scoring in cardiac CT angiography using paired convolutional neural networks. Med Image Anal 2016;34:123–36.

37. de Vos BD, Wolterink JM, Leiner T, et al. Direct Automatic Coronary Calcium Scoring in Cardiac and Chest CT. IEEE Trans Med Imaging 2019;38(9):2127–38.

38. Takx RA, de Jong PA, Leiner T, et al. Automated coronary artery calcification scoring in non-gated chest CT: agreement and reliability. PLoS One 2014;9(3):e91239.

39. Lessmann N, van Ginneken B, Zreik M, et al. Automatic calcium scoring in low-dose chest CT using deep neural networks with dilated convolutions. IEEE Trans Med Imaging 2018;37(2):615–25.

40. Gernaat SAM, van Velzen SGM, Koh V, et al. Automatic quantification of calcifications in the coronary arteries and thoracic aorta on radiotherapy planning CT scans of Western and Asian breast cancer patients. Radiother Oncol 2018;127(3):487–92.

41. Lin A, Dey D, Wong DTL, et al. Perivascular adipose tissue and coronary atherosclerosis: from biology to imaging phenotyping. Curr Atheroscler Rep 2019; 21(12):47.

42. Commandeur F, Goeller M, Razipour A, et al. Fully automated ct quantification of epicardial adipose tissue by deep learning: a multicenter study. Radiol Artif Intell 2019;1(6):e190045.

43. Eisenberg E, McElhinney PA, Commandeur F, et al. Deep learning-based quantification of epicardial adipose tissue volume and attenuation predicts major adverse cardiovascular events in asymptomatic subjects. Circ Cardiovasc Imaging 2020;13(2): e009829.

44. Arbustini E, Narula N, Tavazzi L, et al. The MOGE(S) classification of cardiomyopathy for clinicians. J Am Coll Cardiol 2014;64(3):304–18.

45. Patel AR, Kramer CM. Role of cardiac magnetic resonance in the diagnosis and prognosis of nonischemic cardiomyopathy. JACC Cardiovasc Imaging 2017;10(10 Pt A):1180–93.

46. Augusto JB, Davies RH, Bhuva AN, et al. Diagnosis and risk stratification in hypertrophic cardiomyopathy using machine learning wall thickness measurement: a comparison with human test-retest performance. Lancet Digital Health 2021;3(1):e20–8.

47. Fahmy AS, Neisius U, Chan RH, et al. Three-dimensional deep convolutional neural networks for automated myocardial scar quantification in hypertrophic cardiomyopathy: a multicenter multivendor study. Radiology 2020;294(1):52–60.

48. Ruijsink B, Puyol-Antón E, Oksuz I, et al. Fully automated, quality-controlled cardiac analysis from CMR: validation and large-scale application to characterize cardiac function. JACC: Cardiovasc Imaging 2020;13(3):684–95.

49. Neisius U, El-Rewaidy H, Nakamori S, et al. Radiomic analysis of myocardial native T(1) imaging discriminates between hypertensive heart disease and hypertrophic cardiomyopathy. JACC Cardiovasc Imaging 2019;12(10):1946–54.

50. Satriano A, Afzal Y, Sarim Afzal M, et al. Neural-network-based diagnosis using 3-dimensional myocardial architecture and deformation: demonstration for the differentiation of hypertrophic cardiomyopathy. original research. Front Cardiovasc Med 2020;7:241.

51. Zhou H, Li L, Liu Z, et al. Deep learning algorithm to improve hypertrophic cardiomyopathy mutation prediction using cardiac cine images. Eur Radiol 2021; 31(6):3931–40.

52. Alis D, Guler A, Yergin M, et al. Assessment of ventricular tachyarrhythmia in patients with hypertrophic cardiomyopathy with machine learning-based texture analysis of late gadolinium enhancement cardiac MRI. Diagn Interv Imaging 2020;101(3): 137–46.

53. Shao XN, Sun YJ, Xiao KT, et al. Texture analysis of magnetic resonance T1 mapping with dilated cardiomyopathy: A machine learning approach. Medicine 2018;97(37):e12246.

54. MacGregor RM, Guo A, Masood MF, et al. Machine learning outcome prediction in dilated cardiomyopathy using regional left ventricular multiparametric strain. Ann Biomed Eng 2021;49(2):922–32.

55. Chen R, Lu A, Wang J, et al. Using machine learning to predict one-year cardiovascular events in patients with severe dilated cardiomyopathy. Eur J Radiol 2019;117:178–83.

56. Rocon C, Tabassian M, Tavares de Melo MD, et al. Biventricular imaging markers to predict outcomes in non-compaction cardiomyopathy: a machine learning study. ESC Heart Fail 2020;7(5):2431–9.

57. Ouyang D, He B, Ghorbani A, et al. Video-based AI for beat-to-beat assessment of cardiac function. Nature 2020;580(7802):252–6.

58. Asch FM, Poilvert N, Abraham T, et al. Automated echocardiographic quantification of left ventricular ejection fraction without volume measurements using a machine learning algorithm mimicking a human expert. Circ Cardiovasc Imaging 2019;12(9):e009303.

59. Reddy YNV, Carter RE, Obokata M, et al. A simple, evidence-based approach to help guide diagnosis of heart failure with preserved ejection fraction. Circulation 2018;138(9):861–70.

60. Tabassian M, Sunderji I, Erdei T, et al. Diagnosis of heart failure with preserved ejection fraction: machine learning of spatiotemporal variations in left ventricular deformation. J Am Soc Echocardiogr 2018;31(12):1272–84.e9.

61. Sanchez-Martinez S, Duchateau N, Erdei T, et al. Machine learning analysis of left ventricular function to characterize heart failure with preserved ejection fraction. Circ Cardiovasc Imaging 2018;11(4): e007138.

62. Jing L, Ulloa Cerna AE, Good CW, et al. A machine learning approach to management of heart failure populations. JACC Heart Fail 2020;8(7):578–87.

63. Samad MD, Ulloa A, Wehner GJ, et al. Predicting survival from large echocardiography and electronic health record datasets: optimization with machine learning. JACC: Cardiovasc Imaging 2019;12(4): 681–9.

64. Kwon J-m, Kim K-H, Jeon K-H, et al. Artificial intelligence algorithm for predicting mortality of patients with acute heart failure. PLoS One 2019;14(7): e0219302.

65. Kwon JM, Kim KH, Jeon KH, et al. Deep learning for predicting in-hospital mortality among heart disease patients based on echocardiography. Echocardiography 2019;36(2):213–8.

66. Ulloa Cerna AE, Jing L, Good CW, et al. Deep-learning-assisted analysis of echocardiographic videos improves predictions of all-cause mortality. Nat Biomed Eng 2021;5(6):546–54.

67. Zhang Q, Burrage MK, Lukaschuk E, et al. Towards replacing late gadolinium enhancement with artificial intelligence virtual native enhancement for gadolinium-free cardiovascular magnetic resonance tissue characterization in hypertrophic cardiomyopathy. Circulation 2021. https://doi.org/10.1161/CIRCULATIONAHA.121.054432.

68. Madani A, Ong JR, Tibrewal A, et al. Deep echocardiography: data-efficient supervised and semi-supervised deep learning towards automated diagnosis of cardiac disease. NPJ Digit Med 2018;1(1):59.

69. Zhao M, Liu X, Liu H, et al. Super-resolution of cardiac magnetic resonance images using Laplacian Pyramid based on Generative Adversarial Networks. Comput Med Imaging Graph 2020;80:101698.

70. Diller GP, Vahle J, Radke R, et al. Utility of deep learning networks for the generation of artificial cardiac magnetic resonance images in congenital heart disease. BMC Med Imaging 2020;20(1):113.

71. Gillies RJ, Kinahan PE, Hricak H. Radiomics: images are more than pictures, they are data. Radiology 2016;278(2):563–77.

72. Kagiyama N, Shrestha S, Cho JS, et al. A low-cost texture-based pipeline for predicting myocardial tissue remodeling and fibrosis using cardiac ultrasound. EBioMedicine 2020;54:102726.

73. Kolossváry M, Karády J, Kikuchi Y, et al. Radiomics versus Visual and Histogram-based Assessment to Identify Atheromatous Lesions at Coronary CT Angiography: An ex Vivo Study. Radiology 2019;293(1):89–96.

74. Oikonomou EK, Williams MC, Kotanidis CP, et al. A novel machine learning-derived radiotranscriptomic signature of perivascular fat improves cardiac risk prediction using coronary CT angiography. Eur Heart J 2019;40(43):3529–43.

75. Baessler B, Mannil M, Maintz D, et al. Texture analysis and machine learning of non-contrast T1-weighted MR images in patients with hypertrophic cardiomyopathy-Preliminary results. Eur J Radiol 2018;102:61–7.

76. Larroza A, Lopez-Lereu MP, Monmeneu JV, et al. Texture analysis of cardiac cine magnetic resonance imaging to detect nonviable segments in patients with chronic myocardial infarction. Med Phys 2018;45(4):1471–80.

77. Jobin A, Ienca M, Vayena E. The global landscape of AI ethics guidelines. Nat Machine Intelligence 2019;1(9):389–99.

78. Rigby MJ. Ethical dimensions of using artificial intelligence in health care. AMA J Ethics 2019;21:121–4.

79. Ethics Guidelines for Trustworthy AI (European Commission, 2019). Available at: https://ec.europa.eu/digital-single-market/en/news/ethics-guidelines-trustworthy-ai. Accessed June 29, 2021.

Utilizing Artificial Intelligence to Enhance Health Equity Among Patients with Heart Failure

Amber E. Johnson, MD, MS, MBA[a], LaPrincess C. Brewer, MD, MPH[b],
Melvin R. Echols, MD[c], Sula Mazimba, MD, MPH[d],
Rashmee U. Shah, MD, MS[e], Khadijah Breathett, MD, MS[f],*

KEYWORDS

- Artificial intelligence • Machine learning • Health equity • Racial disparities • Risk prediction
- Guideline-directed therapy • Health services research

KEY POINTS

- Social Determinants of health, bias, and structural racism are major contributors to racial disparities in heart failure.
- Many current forms of artificial intelligence contribute to structural racism via improperly designed and unvalidated models.
- Diversifying the training models for artificial intelligence and the scientific team developing the models may make increase the likelihood of achieving equity in heart failure.

INTRODUCTION

Heart failure (HF) care is inequitable across racial and ethnic populations. Black and Latinx patients have the highest prevalence of HF compared with other racial and ethnic groups,[1] and Black patients have disproportionately higher mortality rates than White patients.[2] Minoritized racial and ethnic populations with HF are less likely to receive evidence-based medications,[3] devices,[4] care by a cardiologist,[5] and heart transplantation.[6] Bias, structural racism, and social determinants of health have been implicated in unequal treatment of patients with HF.[7-10] Multiple strategies are needed to address these pervasive inequalities. This review highlights one important strategy, artificial intelligence (AI).

AI is gaining traction as a means of providing personalized health care in the HF population and is uniquely positioned to enhance the interpretation of heterogeneous clinical data. Patients living with HF may access multiple risk calculators and self-care tools, which are becoming increasingly ubiquitous. Although there are many strengths for broad use of AI, inadequate development and implementation can worsen racial and ethnic disparities in HF. The objectives of this review are to define AI from a health equity lens, describe current use in

Conflict of interest disclosures: None reported.
[a] University of Pittsburgh School of Medicine, Heart and Vascular Institute, Veterans Affairs Pittsburgh Health System, 200 Lothrop Street, Pittsburgh, PA 15213, USA; [b] Division of Preventive Cardiology, Department of Cardiovascular Medicine, Mayo Clinic College of Medicine, 200 First Street SW, Rochester, MN 55905, USA; [c] Division of Cardiovascular Medicine, Morehouse School of Medicine, 720 Westview Drive, Atlanta, GA 30310, USA; [d] Division of Cardiovascular Medicine, Advanced Heart Failure and Transplant Center, University of Virginia, 2nd Floor, 1221 Lee Street, Charlottesville, VA 22903, USA; [e] Division of Cardiovascular Medicine, University of Utah, 30 N 1900 E, Cardiology, 4A100, Salt Lake City, UT 84132, USA; [f] Division of Cardiovascular Medicine, Sarver Heart Center, University of Arizona, 1501 North Campbell Avenue, PO Box 245046, Tucson, AZ 85724, USA
* Corresponding author.
E-mail addresses: kbreathett@shc.arizona.edu; kbreath@iu.edu

Heart Failure Clin 18 (2022) 259–273
https://doi.org/10.1016/j.hfc.2021.11.001
1551-7136/22/© 2021 Elsevier Inc. All rights reserved.

HF, describe the potential strengths and harms in using AI, and offer recommendations for future directions to establish equity in HF.

DEFINITIONS

AI can be conceptualized as (1) rules-based computing—typical "if-then" statements—and (2) machine learning (ML)—where programmed algorithms modify themselves with new information. ML uses so-called deep learning with reliance on statistical principles and reward-based learning to create artificial neural networks or complex connections between bits of information. Therefore, AI can be used for clinical prediction models that make medical diagnoses and prognosticate clinical outcomes.[11]

As the use of AI in health care settings has become more common, so has the complexity of the predictive models. Neural networks use input from a large number of variables to create nonlinear models that expand beyond linear regression models to predict an outcome. Random forest algorithms use branching logic to make decisions about clinical outcomes. Ideally, the resultant models can determine meaningful differences between comparator groups (eg, determining if a patient will have a normal ejection fraction [EF] vs one that is abnormally low). The accuracy of the models to discriminate between groups can be measured in several ways. The C statistic has been the most widely reported measure of model discrimination for cardiovascular risk prediction.[12] On aggregate, the available data suggest that ML is a valid tool for risk prediction.

However, using AI for risk estimation also has some limitations. Biases are systematic misinterpretations of data, processes, or decision-making. Such systematic inaccuracies have detrimental effects on outcome reliability, validity, and equity.[13] There are 2 main types of bias to think of: (1) algorithmic bias and (2) social bias or unfairness. Regarding the first type, AI developers who create models and supervise ML algorithms will try to minimize statistical error when programming a model. Yet, social bias may be less readily detected. Nevertheless, policymakers and national agencies are beginning to prioritize the detection and prevention of social bias in AI. Some clinical enterprises believe that multimodal data and so-called learning health systems can assist in the delivery of unbiased care.[14] In addition, the National Institutes of Health are working to understand how to build across communities for data generation projects based on ethical principles.[15]

CURRENT USE

Some of the earliest visible work in this field was geared heavily toward minoritized racial/ethnic populations from socioeconomically disadvantaged communities. In 2011, the Parkland Health and Hospital System, which serves communities with low economic resources around Dallas, Texas, faced sanctions from the Center for Medicaid and Medicare Services for high readmission rates and poor outcomes.[16] Around that time, a team of clinician-scientists harnessed electronic medical record (EMR) data to predict patients at increased risk of 30-day readmission and death. The internal model yielded a C statistical of 0.86 for mortality and 0.72 for readmission, an improvement over pre-existing models at the time.[17] In this study, 62.1% of patients were Black race. In a follow-up, prospective study, the team was able to demonstrate a small, but measurable, reduction in readmissions by using the EMR-based model to redirect health system resources.[18]

Despite a robust number of HF trials, most studies on ML methods either lack a diverse racial and ethnic population or fail to disclose race and ethnicity of the patients (**Table 1**). Thus, we are unable to determine if the results are applicable to racially diverse groups. This issue is particularly relevant to ML because the data are often observational in nature and are prone to algorithmic bias, which could have a greater impact on model accuracy for minoritized groups. In addition, much of the work has been done outside of the United States, with different social constructs surrounding race and health care delivery. As a notable addition to the literature, Segar and colleagues recently found that ML models derived with race used as a covariate have inferior performance compared with race-specific models.[19]

AI models are only as reliable as the data from which they are built, and the statistical assessment of the models is subject to limitations. For example, the C statistical is derived from the model's sensitivity and specificity and can be insensitive to changes in absolute risk.[12] Therefore, in the available literature, the C statistics comparing AI models to standard risk prediction models may not fully convey clinically meaningful results or may overestimate the models' clinical relevance. In addition to the questionable improvement over traditional approaches, the literature illustrates that AI and ML prediction models require large amounts of readily available data to train the algorithms. Subsequent implementation of AI into routine health care delivery can also pose a logistical concern.

In the conduct of HF AI studies, researchers have linked large registry data sets with insurance

Table 1
Example studies that apply machine learning to heart failure–specific clinical questions

Study	Outcome	Race/Ethnicity Distribution
Prediction		
Wu et al,[69] 2021	Predict HF among patients with hypertension from a broad range of EMR data; An 11-variable combination was considered most valuable for predicting outcomes using the ML approach. The C statistical for identifying patients with composite end points was 0.757 (95% CI, 0.660–0.854) for the ML model	Not reported
Maragatham and Devi,[70] 2019	Predict HF by applying a RNN to EMR data; C statistical 0.70–0.80	Not reported
Choi et al,[71] 2017	Predict incident HF by applying a neural network to EMR data; C statistical for the RNN model was 0.777, compared with C statistical for logistic regression (0.747), MLP with 1 hidden layer (0.765), SVM (0.743), and KNN (0.730). When using an 18-mo observation window, the C statistical for the RNN model increased to 0.883 and was significantly higher than the 0.834 C statistical for the best of the baseline methods (MLP)	Not reported
Segar et al,[72] 2019	Predict HF among patients with diabetes by applying random forest to the ACCORD data, with validation in ALLHAT; RSF models demonstrated better discrimination than the best performing Cox-based method (C statistical 0.77 [95% CI, 0.75–0.80] vs 0.73 [95% CI, 0.70–0.76], respectively) and had acceptable calibration (Hosmer-Lemeshow statistical $\chi^2 = 9.63$, $P = .29$) in the internal validation data set). In the external validation cohort, the RSF-based risk prediction model and the WATCH-DM risk score performed well with good discrimination (C statistical = 0.74 and 0.70, respectively), acceptable calibration ($P < .20$ for both)	18.5% Black in training; 38% in ALLHAT

(continued on next page)

Table 1
(continued)

Study	Outcome	Race/Ethnicity Distribution
Segar et al,[19] 2021	HF risk prediction models were developed separately for Black (JHS cohort) and White participants (ARIC cohort). The derivation cohorts were randomly split into a training (50%) and testing (50%) data set. The results showed that race-specific ML models can predict 10-y risk of incident HF among cohorts of White (n = 7858 in ARIC, C-index = 0.89) and Black patients (n = 4141 in JHS, C-index = 0.88).	n = 4141 Black in the training set; n = 2821 Black in the validation set
Diagnosis		
Tabassian et al,[73] 2018	Discriminate HFpEF patients from others using strain data from stress echocardiography; 51% accuracy	Not reported
Agliari et al,[74] 2020	Diagnose HF using heart rate variability derived from 24-h Holter monitors	Not reported
Farmakis et al,[75] 2016	Diagnose HFrEF using urinary proteomic evaluation; support vector machine-based classifier that was successfully applied to a test set of 25 HFrEF patients and 33 controls, achieving 84% sensitivity and 91% specificity	Not reported
Rossing et al,[76] 2016	Diagnose HFrEF using urinary proteomic evaluation; HFrEF103 very accurately (C statistical = 0.972) discriminated between HFrEF patients (N = 94, sensitivity = 93.6%)	Not reported
Cho et al,[77] 2021	Diagnose ejection fraction <41% using 12-lead ECG; C statistical 0.91 in the training	Not reported
Attia et al,[78] 2019	Diagnose ejection fraction <36% using 12-lead ECG; C statistical 0.93 in the validation set	Not reported

(continued on next page)

Table 1 (continued)		
Study	**Outcome**	**Race/Ethnicity Distribution**
Phenotypes		
Zhang et al,[79] 2018	Extract NYHA class using natural language processing of clinical text from the EMR; The best machine learning method was a random forest with n-gram features (F-measure: 93.78%).	Not reported
Omar et al,[80] 2018	Estimate LV fill pressure from speckle tracking echocardiography; predictive ability of ML model for elevated LVFP (C statistical: training cohort: 0.847, testing cohort:0.868)	Not reported
Cikes et al,[31] 2019	Unsupervised machine learning algorithm to cluster MADI-CRT trial participants into 4 phenogroups, 2 of which were associated with CRT response	Reported as 91% White race
Feeny et al,[81] 2019	Use ML to predict EF improvement among CRT recipients, combining 9 features from ECG, echo, and other clinical characteristics; ML demonstrated better response prediction than guidelines (C statistical, 0.70 vs 0.65; $P = .012$) and greater discrimination of event-free survival (concordance index, 0.61 vs 0.56; $P < .001$).	Not reported
Hirata et al,[82] 2021	Predict wedge pressure >17 mm Hg by applying deep learning algorithm to a chest x-ray; C statistical = 0.77 for DL model	Not reported
Shah et al,[29] 2015	An unsupervised machine learning algorithm to cluster 397 patients with HFpEF into 3 distinct phenogroups; The mean age was 65 ± 12 y; 62% were women	39% Black participants

(continued on next page)

Table 1
(continued)

Study	Outcome	Race/Ethnicity Distribution
Prognosis		
Hearn et al,[83] 2018	Predict initiation of mechanical circulatory support, listing for heart transplantation or mortality using cardiopulmonary exercise test data; neural network incorporating breath-by-breath data achieving the best performance (C statistical = 0.842)	Not reported
Kwon et al,[84] 2019	Use echocardiography data to predict in-hospital mortality; DL (C statistical: 0.913 AUPRC: 0.351) significantly outperformed MAGGIC (C statistical: 0.806, C statistical: 0.154) and GWTG-HF (C statistical: 0.783, C statistical: 0.285) for HF during external validation	Not reported
Przewlocka-Kosmala et al,[85] 2019	Predict composite end point of CV hospitalization or death and HF hospitalization using stress echocardiography, CPET, serum galectin-3, and BNP using hierarchical clustering	Not reported
Allam et al,[86] 2019	Predict 30-d readmission among HF patients by applying neural networks to administrative claims data; C statistics 0.642 at best	Not reported
Frizzell et al,[20] 2017	Predict 30-d readmission among HF patients enrolled in GWTG-HF, linked with Medicare; For the tree-augmented naive Bayesian network, random forest, gradient-boosted, logistic regression, and least absolute shrinkage and selection operator models, C statistics for the validation sets were similar: 0.618, 0.607, 0.614, 0.624, and 0.618, respectively	Found in supplement (10% Black, 4.5% Hispanic, and 1.3% Asian)

(continued on next page)

Table 1
(continued)

Study	Outcome	Race/Ethnicity Distribution
Desai et al,[21] 2020	Predict all-cause mortality, HF hospitalization, top cost decile, and home days loss >25% using EMR linked to Medicare; GBM was best but no better than logistic regression; (C statistics for logistic regression based on claims-only predictors: mortality, 0.724; 95% CI, 0.705–0.744; HF hospitalization, 0.707; 95% CI, 0.676–0.737; high cost, 0.734; 95% CI, 0.703–0.764; and home days loss claims only, 0.781; 95% CI, 0.764–0.798; C statistics for GBM: mortality, 0.727; 95% CI, 0.708–0.747; HF hospitalization, 0.745; 95% CI, 0.718–0.772; high cost, 0.733; 95% CI, 0.703–0.763; and home days loss, 0.790; 95% CI, 0.773–0.807	5.1% Black participants
Angraal et al,[22] 2020	Predict death and HF hospitalization in the TOPCAT trial. The RF was the best performing model with a mean C-statistic of 0.72 (95% CI, 0.69–0.75) for predicting mortality (Brier score, 0.17), and 0.76 (95% CI, 0.71–0.81) for HF hospitalization (Brier score, 0.19)	78.3% White participants
Tokodi et al,[87] 2020	Predict mortality among patients undergoing CRT implantation; C statistical for 5-y mortality was 0.803, compared with 0.693 for the next best performing model	Not reported

Abbreviations: CI, confidence interval; CV, cardiovascular; HFpEF, HF with preserved ejection fraction; KNN, K-nearest neighbor; LV, left ventricle; MLP, multilayer perceptron; RNN, recurrent neural network; SVM, support vector machine.

claims data to predict clinical outcomes. Frizell and colleagues used the American Heart Association Get With the Guidelines Heart Failure (GWTG-HF) registry linked with Medicare inpatient data to develop ML models to predict readmission within 30 days after discharge of an index HF hospitalization.[20] Discrimination was suboptimal, with C statistics ranging from 0.607 to 0.624; ML models performed no better than logistic regression.[20] Similarly, Desai and colleagues developed models to predict mortality and HF hospitalization using health system data linked to Medicare.[21] They, too, found that AI models performed no better

than linear regression models, with C statistics ranging from 0.700 to 0.778 for both outcomes.[21] A post hoc analysis of the TOPCAT (Treatment of Preserved Cardiac Function Heart Failure with an Aldosterone Antagonist) trial had slightly more promising results. Angraal and colleagues compared 5 different methods to predict mortality and HF hospitalization.[22] The random forest model performed best, with a C statistical of 0.72 (95% confidence interval [CI], 0.69–0.75) for mortality and 0.76 (95% CI, 0.71–0.81) for hospitalization.[22] These models, however, cannot be applied broadly because they require data that were collected as part of a clinical trial, outside of routine health care delivery.

The current data show that AI is feasible in clinical trials, but more pragmatic studies are needed to show clinical effectiveness, especially among diverse populations. To date, very few models have been tested prospectively. Fortunately, this landscape is changing. Medical journals are encouraging prespecification of methods and outcomes, even for retrospective analyses. Through this process, journal editors could require reporting of population demographics and diversity. Because clinical inequities abound in a myriad of patient encounters across the spectrum of the health care system (research and development, clinical practice and population health),[23] the available data sets from which AI models are trained may be prone to the perpetuation of social bias.[24,25] For these and other reasons, there are growing calls for the judicious implementation of AI models that are grounded in relational ethics that prioritize justice and promote equity.[26]

HEALTH DISPARITIES AND ARTIFICIAL INTELLIGENCE IN HF CARE

Despite major advances in diagnostic and therapeutic modalities for HF, health care disparities and inequities have persisted.[27,28] AI models could aid in the delivery of quality care by enhancing diagnosis, categorization, and identification of patient groups at risk of adverse events, medication nonadherence, and HF readmission.[29–31] Importantly, AI holds promise in the identification of distinct phenotypes of cardiovascular disorders for which racially diverse populations suffer disparate outcomes.[32] For example, prediction models for HF with preserved ejection fraction (HFpEF) show that AI models can cluster patients into distinct groups to tailor specific therapies.[29] A precise, individualized approach to patients' needs potentially combines sociodemographic characteristics, phenotype, genotype, and biomarkers to determine clinical care.[33] In this sense, the intersection of precision medicine and AI holds tremendous promise for alleviating health disparities, such as underutilization of guideline-directed medical therapy (GDMT).[34,35]

AI models can enhance clinical productivity by using the existing, available data to provide timely diagnosis and avoid cognitive bias in clinical encounters.[36–38] A recent study using an ML model to predict HF prognosis outperformed existing HF risk models.[39] Other potential applications of AI include the use of decision aids, prompting clinicians to use GDMT. This approach has great potential for enhancing uptake in the use of GDMT, which still remains suboptimal, as evidenced

from a contemporary real-world HF registry.[40] For example, guideline-recommended, adjunctive therapy for HF in patients with African ancestry with hydralazine and isosorbide dinitrate has been underutilized in Europe.[41] These results parallel similar findings in the United States where utilization of cardiac resynchronization therapies and advanced HF therapy uptake among Black patients remains suboptimal compared with White patients.[6,42] A clinical trial, TRANSFORM-HFrEF (NCT04872959), will soon be underway, testing whether the use of ML prompted GDMT recommendations from EMR would lead to greater adoption of GDMT over standard care. The results of this trial may shape future directions in the use of ML for adjusting GDMT in patients with HF.

At the population level, efforts to enhance health equity could incorporate AI to decipher the heterogeneity among patients with HF. Improvements in HF survival have been attributed to pharmacologic and nonpharmacologic therapies, which have demonstrated substantial benefit at a population level.[35,43] However, some subpopulations of HF patients have not derived benefits and, in some cases, have experienced harm.[44] These discrepancies can be attributed to heterogeneity in patient populations and variations in pathophysiological processes of HF. Such variations may include social determinants of health as well as "-omics" (ie, - genomics, pharmacogenomics, epigenomics, proteomics, metabolomics, and microbiomics). Advances in ML techniques can help integrate all these complex applications in clinical practice.[29,43,45]

AI, ML, and deep learning methodologies are prime for further study of the associations between race and HF outcomes. Race, a social construct, should be distinguished from ancestry-informative genetic markers. Race is also confounded with other social stratifications such as income level, educational attainment, location of residence, and environmental exposures.[46,47] AI can accelerate the development of predictive models as tools to overcome race-based health disparities. So long as future models use ethnic diversity in genomics biorepositories with ancestry-matched controls, researchers will be able to address relevant genomic information in light of their social and cultural implications.[48]

POTENTIAL HARMS OF ARTIFICIAL INTELLIGENCE IN HF CARE

AI has drawn recent criticism for egregious failures of facial recognition technology.[49,50] In 2015, a popular online search engine launched a photograph application with automated tagging capabilities to assist users in organizing uploaded images.

Unfortunately, the automated facial recognition software labeled a photograph of Black people as "gorillas."[51,52] Although the company apologized for this error, the incident serves as an example of one of the many forms of racism demonstrated via AI technology. In 2018, a study evaluated 3 different facial recognition platforms used by law enforcement agencies to find criminal suspects or missing children.[52] The investigators analyzed a diverse sample of 1270 people. The programs misidentified up to 35% of dark-skinned women as men, compared with a top error rate for light-skinned men of only 0.8%.[50] AI utilization for law enforcement exemplifies harm concerning the strained social justice of racially minoritized groups in society. The selection of training data sets derived from homogenous populations will continue to perpetuate algorithmic biases against more diverse populations. Thus, developing a diverse training data set is crucial to producing reliable assumptions with adequate generalizability.

In addition to generalizability, efficacy remains a major concern when applying AI in nonresearch settings, and AI could cause harm when research prototypes are distributed more broadly. For example, retinal detection software was developed to diagnose diabetic retinopathy. However, tests in rural India demonstrated the challenges of transferring such technology into the clinical setting.[53] The software failed to make a diagnosis because of the poor-quality images available in resource-limited settings. Thus, even in populations with minimal racial variation, AI has limitations of algorithmic or procedural bias that can prohibit adequate health care utility.

Furthermore, AI-derived assumptions can lead to data misinterpretation when the models are applied to broader clinical scenarios than the data sets upon which they were built.[51] In a study by Obermeyer and colleagues, investigators evaluated a sample of insured patients with medical comorbidities. The cohort included 6079 patients who self-identified as Black race and 43,539 patients who self-identified as White race with over 11,929 and 88,080 patient-years of data, respectively.[25] The investigators used AI to determine a predictive model of health care needs based on the number of active chronic conditions, comorbidity score, and race. The final algorithm predicted health care costs as a proxy for health care needs. However, race-based disparities in access to care are a major contributor to less care and less spending for Black patients compared with White patients. As a result, illness was not a significant contributor to the model, despite its clinical significance. Although health care cost can be considered an effective proxy for health in some circumstances, this AI-derived proxy introduced substantial clinical limitations for Black patients.[25] If AI-derived algorithms of this nature were to be used in determining resource allocation, disproportionally affected HF populations would likely have worsened outcomes.

Implicit bias, or the unconscious process of associating assumptions or attitudes toward populations of people, can influence individual decision-making for people and neural networks alike.[9,54–57] Such implicit biases within AI-derived models form the foundation for structural or systemic biases, resulting in racial discrimination. Even with good intentions and diverse data, there are several socially biased misinterpretations of the results that could lead to harm. Using subjective rather than objective data is a known factor in socially biased decisions that adversely impact minoritized patient populations.[7,10] Developers and researchers must be deliberate in the design phase of any AI-driven project and be aware that any outcome may likely have blind spots.[51] Investigators must be well-versed in the intricacies of AI research and include a diverse group of developers and collaborators before clinical, political, or legal implementation.

RECOMMENDATIONS AND FUTURE DIRECTIONS
Addressing Known Biases and Structural Racism

Although it is impossible to address unknown problems, a critical analysis of health inequity requires an intentional focus on disempowered and marginalized populations[58,59] when programming and training AI algorithms (**Fig. 1**). For example, in a national study of approximately 500 hospitals, patient race was associated with the likelihood of receiving care by a cardiologist when hospitalized in an intensive care setting for a primary diagnosis of HF.[5] White patients were 42% more likely to receive care by a cardiologist than Black patients.[5] Black men were the least likely to receive care by a cardiologist despite having increased survival benefit with care by a cardiologist.[5] Similar findings were observed in a retrospective cohort study of 1967 patients receiving care at an academic medical center.[60] The study revealed biases that were hidden in plain sight: Black and Latinx patients were less likely to be admitted to an inpatient cardiology service (adjusted relative risk [RR] 0.91 [95% CI, 0.84–0.98; P = .019]; RR 0.83 [95% CI, 0.72–0.97; P = .017], respectively). This disparity led to higher 30-day readmission rates among

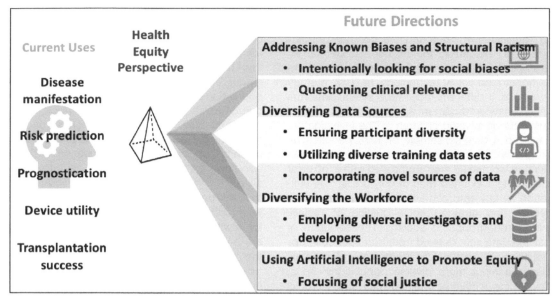

Fig. 1. Current AI use and future directions (central illustration). AI can predict differential HF outcomes. Future directions will lead to underlying pathophysiological mechanisms, developing novel equitable therapies, and improving the performance of new clinical approaches. By incorporating intentional ethical principles into data science, the field is expected to address known biases and structural racism, diversify data sources, diversify the workforce, and prioritize opportunities that promote equity.

Black and Latinx patients, further perpetuating existing poor HF outcomes in these groups. One of the strongest predictors of admission to the inpatient cardiology service was having an outpatient cardiologist, which unfortunately Black and Latinx patients were less likely to have. The institution has admirably acknowledged this form of structural racism and has plans to implement strategies to look beyond race as a biologic variable by addressing the social determinants of health.[61]

To further this aim, the deployment of a fair allocation-focused AI strategy could potentially optimize quality of care and reduce and ultimately eliminate inequities in hospital readmissions for Black and Latinx patients with HF. Equal allocation mechanisms through use of the EMR could assist in triaging these patient populations to appropriate specialized care as well as securing adequate outpatient follow-up (eg, cardiovascular specialist, cardiac rehabilitation) and community-based resources (eg, medication vouchers, employment opportunities, social support, etc)—potentially correcting this bias. Incorporation of the social determinants of health variables (eg, income, insurance status, food, housing insecurity, etc) into ML algorithms to not primarily rely on race could improve the accuracy of their "eligibility" predictions or detection and the fairness of decisions to ultimately allocate interventions, services, and treatments to patients who need them most.[62]

In addition to approaching clinical questions through a health equity lens, known biases can also be prevented using supervised algorithms. Unsupervised algorithms (eg, support vector machines) use statistical learning models and assume naturally occurring subsets of data that behave differently yet predictably across populations and clinical scenarios. Some data, such as race, may not behave as "predicted." Thus, the intrinsic structure within HF patient phenotypic data must be re-evaluated retrospectively and prospectively for predicting treatment outcomes, guiding clinical care, and developing further research questions.[29]

Diversifying Data Sources

AI models are only as reliable as the data from which they are built, and the statistical assessment of the models is subject to limitations. The selection of training data sets derived from homogenous populations will continue to perpetuate algorithmic biases against more diverse populations. Thus, developing a diverse training data set is crucial to producing reliable assumptions with adequate generalizability.

Diversity drives excellence and creative problem-solving.[63] From the outset, ensuring the use of diverse patient population databases and the incorporation of diverse data scientists are key; not doing so can deepen health and health care disparities.[64] Telemedicine and mobile health care delivery, coupled with sophisticated algorithms, could change the way we deliver care,[65] particularly if the algorithms can direct precise treatments to the patients who would benefit most.[66]

Diversifying the Workforce

Workforce diversity can lead to improved patient outcomes and enhance creativity and innovation. It should be a priority to include researchers and data scientists who are representative of diverse patients; this may help develop effective and culturally relevant tools to tackle health inequities.[63] One of the valuable assets of diverse teams is the ability to create algorithms that are based on the sociocultural and environmental contexts that better contribute to our understanding of disease processes, management, and outcomes. Diversity in thought and experience on the team should include individuals with expertise on how disparities contextually arise. These team members can work collaboratively with AI developers to recognize and address any inscribed biases within models.[13] This may help address AI concerns expanding beyond health care to education and the restorative justice system.

Along those same lines, centrality of the patient and community are essential. Community partnerships and diverse stakeholder engagement[67] may increase data diversity, research participation, and fulfill the ethical responsibility to understand the lived experiences of patients with HF. This may help develop contextually informed solutions to provide patients with equitable and quality care. Incorporation of preferences and perspectives from underrepresented minoritized groups may lead to the creation of more meaningful AI tools at the individual, health care provider, health systems, and community levels.

Using AI to Promote Equity

With purposeful clinical and ethical insight, disadvantaged populations and minoritized individuals living with HF can achieve equitable health outcomes. A deliberate objective should be to prioritize those who will be the ultimate beneficiaries of the technology.[13] Rajkomar and colleagues proposed 3 central axes for distributive justice with ML: equal performance, equal patient outcomes, and equal resource allocation.[58] As a case example, Noseworthy and colleagues conducted a retrospective cohort analysis to determine whether a deep learning algorithm to detect low left ventricular EF (LVEF) using 12-lead electrocardiograms varied by race and ethnicity.[68] The

model had previously been derived from and validated in a relatively homogenous population. The analysis demonstrated consistent and optimal performance to detect low LVEF across a range of racial and ethnic subgroups (Non-Hispanic White [N = 44,524, C statistical = 0.931], Asian [N = 557, C statistical = 0.961], Black/African American [N = 651, C statistical = 0.937], Hispanic/Latinx [N = 331, C statistical = 0.937], and American Indian/Alaskan Native [N = 223, C statistical = 0.938]).[68] After determining equal performance, the next step would be to ensure that the ML model is of equal benefit to all patient groups. This should include comprehensive analyses of key patient outcomes (not solely diagnostic outputs) or narrowing of outcome disparities. If disparate outcomes are detected in the development phase, then the model should be revised, repaired, and reanalyzed in a more heterogenous population before deployment for widespread use.

It is essential to note that, although AI can be used to predict differential outcomes, future directions must move beyond mere risk stratification. AI should be used to understand underlying pathophysiological mechanisms, develop specific therapies, and improve the performance of new clinical approaches.[29] Moreover, AI should be used to uncover and address the social and systemic barriers leading to health disparities. It may be necessary to center around previously marginalized groups to model approaches that will overcome disparities in care.[13] Algorithmic systems never emerge in a social, historical, or political vacuum, so by incorporating intentional ethical principles into data science, AI could "learn" to detect and address inequity (see **Fig. 1**).[26]

SUMMARY

When executed with an intentional focus on social justice, AI, ML, and deep learning tools have the potential to enhance equity in racially diverse populations of people with HF. Diverse groups of investigators, developers, and health systems will need to work in concert to create the best environments for equitable AI models. Important variables such as self-identified race must be included in data sets and in the EMR so that they will be considered in analyses that call for social constructs. In addition, genetic admixture data may be used to more precisely evaluate the role of ancestry in clinical outcomes. To best harness, the power of large data sets, race, social determinants of health, and genomic variants will need to become a part of the health systems' EMR. Then, as the models are developed, care must be taken to evaluate the results to ensure that the data have clinical relevance for the populations of interest. Future directions in the field of AI for HF should include addressing known biases, structural racism, diversifying data sources, diversifying the workforce, and finding opportunities that continue to promote equity.

CLINICS CARE POINTS

Before using clinical risk calculators, consider the following:

1. Has this calculator been validated in diverse racial and ethnic populations?
2. Does this calculator contribute to biased decision-making or structural racism?
3. How can I tailor my care plan to address bias, structural racism, and social determinants of health?

SOURCES OF FUNDING

Dr K. Breathett has research funding from National Heart, Lung, and Blood Institute (NHLBI) K01HL142848, R56HL159216, R25HL126146 subaward 11692sc, L30HL148881; and Women as One Escalator Award. Dr L.C. Brewer was supported by the American Heart Association-Amos Medical Faculty Development Program (Grant No. 19AMFDP35040005), NCATS (NCATS, CTSA Grant No. KL2 TR002379), the National Institutes of Health (NIH)/National Institute on Minority Health and Health Disparities (NIMHD) (Grant No. 1 R21 MD013490–01), and the Centers for Disease Control and Prevention (CDC) (Grant No. CDC-DP18-1817) during the implementation of this work. Its contents are solely the responsibility of the authors and do not necessarily represent the official views of NCATS, NIH, or CDC. The funding bodies had no role in study design; in the collection, analysis, and interpretation of data; writing of the article; and in the decision to submit the article for publication. Dr R.U. Shah has research support from the Doris Duke Charitable Foundation and the Women as One Escalator Award.

REFERENCES

1. Virani SS, Alonso A, Aparicio HJ, et al. Heart Disease and Stroke Statistics-2021 Update: A Report From the American Heart Association. Circulation 2021;143(8):e254–743.
2. Glynn P, Lloyd-Jones DM, Feinstein MJ, et al. Disparities in cardiovascular mortality related to heart failure in the United States. J Am Coll Cardiol 2019;73(18):2354–5.
3. Chan PS, Oetgen WJ, Buchanan D, et al. Cardiac performance measure compliance in outpatients: the American College of Cardiology and National Cardiovascular Data Registry's PINNACLE (Practice Innovation And Clinical Excellence) program. J Am Coll Cardiol 2010;56(1):8–14.
4. Farmer SA, Kirkpatrick JN, Heidenreich PA, et al. Ethnic and racial disparities in cardiac resynchronization therapy. Heart Rhythm 2009;6(3):325–31.
5. Breathett K, Liu WG, Allen LA, et al. African Americans are less likely to receive care by a cardiologist during an intensive care unit admission for heart failure. JACC Heart Fail 2018;6(5):413–20.
6. Breathett K, Knapp SM, Carnes M, et al. Imbalance in heart transplant to heart failure mortality ratio among African American, Hispanic, and White Patients. Circulation 2021;143(24):2412–4.
7. Breathett K, Yee E, Pool N, et al. Does race influence decision making for advanced heart failure therapies? J Am Heart Assoc 2019;8(22):e013592.
8. Breathett K, Jones J, Lum HD, et al. Factors related to physician clinical decision-making for African-American and hispanic patients: a qualitative meta-synthesis. J Racial Ethn Health Disparities 2018;5(6):1215–29.
9. Nayak A, Hicks AJ, Morris AA. Understanding the complexity of heart failure risk and treatment in black patients. Circ Heart Fail 2020;13(8):e007264.
10. Breathett K, Yee E, Pool N, et al. Association of gender and race with allocation of advanced heart failure therapies. JAMA Netw Open 2020;3(7):e2011044.
11. What is Artificial Intelligence (AI)? The University of Queensland. Available at: https://qbi.uq.edu.au/brain/intelligent-machines/what-artificial-intelligence-ai. Accessed March 17, 2021.
12. Lloyd-Jones DM. Cardiovascular risk prediction: basic concepts, current status, and future directions. Circulation 2010;121(15):1768–77.
13. Pot M, Kieusseyan N, Prainsack B. Not all biases are bad: equitable and inequitable biases in machine learning and radiology. Insights Imaging 2021;12(1):13.
14. Three Pittsburgh Institutions. One goal. Pittsburgh, Pennsylvania: The Pittsburgh Health Data Alliance; 2021. Available at: https://healthdataalliance.com/partners/. Accessed June 13, 2021.
15. NIH. Bridge to Artificial Intelligence (Bridge2AI). Common Fund. Available at: https://commonfund.nih.gov/bridge2ai. Accessed June 13, 2021.
16. Moukheiber Z. Can Algorithms Save Parkland Hospital? Forbes Magazine. 2012. Available at: https://www.forbes.com/sites/zinamoukheiber/2012/12/28/can-algorithms-save-parkland-hospital/?sh=1717ab4259f1. Accessed May 3, 2021.
17. Amarasingham R, Moore BJ, Tabak YP, et al. An automated model to identify heart failure patients at risk for

30-day readmission or death using electronic medical record data. Med Care 2010;48(11):981–8.

18. Amarasingham R, Patel PC, Toto K, et al. Allocating scarce resources in real-time to reduce heart failure readmissions: a prospective, controlled study. BMJ Qual Saf 2013;22(12):998–1005.

19. Segar MW, Jaeger BC, Patel KV, et al. Development and validation of machine learning-based race-specific models to predict 10-year risk of heart failure: a multicohort analysis. Circulation 2021;143(24):2370–83.

20. Frizzell JD, Liang L, Schulte PJ, et al. Prediction of 30-day all-cause readmissions in patients hospitalized for heart failure: comparison of machine learning and other statistical approaches. JAMA Cardiol 2017;2(2):204–9.

21. Desai RJ, Wang SV, Vaduganathan M, et al. Comparison of machine learning methods with traditional models for use of administrative claims with electronic medical records to predict heart failure outcomes. JAMA Netw Open 2020;3(1):e1918962.

22. Angraal S, Mortazavi BJ, Gupta A, et al. Machine learning prediction of mortality and hospitalization in heart failure with preserved ejection fraction. JACC Heart Fail 2020;8(1):12–21.

23. Johnson KW, Torres Soto J, Glicksberg BS, et al. Artificial intelligence in cardiology. J Am Coll Cardiol 2018;71(23):2668–79.

24. Char DS, Shah NH, Magnus D. Implementing machine learning in health care - addressing ethical challenges. N Engl J Med 2018;378(11):981–3.

25. Obermeyer Z, Powers B, Vogeli C, et al. Dissecting racial bias in an algorithm used to manage the health of populations. Science 2019;366(6464):447–53.

26. Birhane A. Algorithmic injustice: a relational ethics approach. Patterns (N Y) 2021;2(2):100205.

27. Churchwell K, Elkind MSV, Benjamin RM, et al. Call to action: structural racism as a fundamental driver of health disparities: a presidential advisory from the American Heart Association. Circulation 2020;142(24):e454–68.

28. Mwansa H, Lewsey S, Mazimba S, et al. Racial/ethnic and gender disparities in heart failure with reduced ejection fraction. Curr Heart Fail Rep 2021;18(2):41–51.

29. Shah SJ, Katz DH, Selvaraj S, et al. Phenomapping for novel classification of heart failure with preserved ejection fraction. Circulation 2015;131(3):269–79.

30. Awan SE, Sohel F, Sanfilippo FM, et al. Machine learning in heart failure: ready for prime time. Curr Opin Cardiol 2018;33(2):190–5.

31. Cikes M, Sanchez-Martinez S, Claggett B, et al. Machine learning-based phenogrouping in heart failure to identify responders to cardiac resynchronization therapy. Eur J Heart Fail 2019;21(1):74–85.

32. Pandey A, Omar W, Ayers C, et al. Sex and race differences in lifetime risk of heart failure with preserved ejection fraction and heart failure with reduced ejection fraction. Circulation 2018;137(17):1814–23.

33. Jameson JL, Longo DL. Precision medicine–personalized, problematic, and promising. N Engl J Med 2015;372(23):2229–34.

34. Tat E, Bhatt DL, Rabbat MG. Addressing bias: artificial intelligence in cardiovascular medicine. Lancet Digit Health 2020;2(12):e635–6.

35. Maddox TM, Januzzi JL Jr, Allen LA, et al. 2021 Update to the 2017 ACC expert consensus decision pathway for optimization of heart failure treatment: answers to 10 pivotal issues about heart failure with reduced ejection fraction: a Report of the American College of Cardiology Solution Set Oversight Committee. J Am Coll Cardiol 2021;77(6):772–810.

36. Berner ES, Webster GD, Shugerman AA, et al. Performance of four computer-based diagnostic systems. N Engl J Med 1994;330(25):1792–6.

37. Lopez-Jimenez F, Attia Z, Arruda-Olson AM, et al. Artificial intelligence in cardiology: present and future. Mayo Clin Proc 2020;95(5):1015–39.

38. Ng K, Steinhubl SR, deFilippi C, et al. Early detection of heart failure using electronic health records: practical implications for time before diagnosis, data diversity, data quantity, and data density. Circ Cardiovasc Qual Outcomes 2016;9(6):649–58.

39. Adler ED, Voors AA, Klein L, et al. Improving risk prediction in heart failure using machine learning. Eur J Heart Fail 2020;22(1):139–47.

40. Greene SJ, Butler J, Albert NM, et al. Medical therapy for heart failure with reduced ejection fraction: the CHAMP-HF registry. J Am Coll Cardiol 2018;72(4):351–66.

41. Brewster LM. Underuse of hydralazine and isosorbide dinitrate for heart failure in patients of African ancestry: a cross-European survey. ESC Heart Fail 2019;6(3):487–98.

42. Breathett K, Allen LA, Helmkamp L, et al. Temporal trends in contemporary use of ventricular assist devices by race and ethnicity. Circ Heart Fail 2018;11(8):e005008.

43. Cresci S, Pereira NL, Ahmad F, et al. Heart failure in the era of precision medicine: a scientific statement from the American Heart Association. Circ Genom Precis Med 2019;12(10):458–85.

44. Ginsburg GS, Phillips KA. Precision medicine: from science to value. Health Aff (Millwood) 2018;37(5):694–701.

45. Cheng S, Shah SH, Corwin EJ, et al. Potential Impact and Study Considerations of metabolomics in cardiovascular health and disease: a scientific statement From the American Heart Association. Circ Cardiovasc Genet 2017;10(2):e1–13.

46. LaVeist TA. Disentangling race and socioeconomic status: a key to understanding health inequalities. J Urban Health 2005;82(2 Suppl 3):iii26–34.

47. Breathett K, Spatz ES, Kramer DB, et al. The groundwater of racial and ethnic disparities research: a statement from circulation: cardiovascular quality and outcomes. Circ Cardiovasc Qual Outcomes 2021;14(2):e007868.

48. Mensah GA, Jaquish C, Srinivas P, et al. Emerging concepts in precision medicine and cardiovascular diseases in racial and ethnic minority populations. Circ Res 2019;125(1):7–13.

49. Han H, Otto C, Liu X, et al. Demographic estimation from face images: human vs. machine performance. IEEE Trans Pattern Anal Mach Intell 2015;37(6): 1148–61.

50. Buolamwini J, Gebru T. Gender Shades: Intersectional Accuracy Disparities in Commercial Gender Classification. Proceedings of the 1st Conference on Fairness, Accountability and Transparency; 2018; Proceedings of Machine Learning Research. Available at: https:// proceedings.mlr.press/v81/buolamwini18a.html.

51. Fawcett A. Understanding racial bias in machine learning algorithms. 2020. Available at: https://www. educative.io/blog/racial-bias-machine-learning-algorithms. Accessed May 9, 2021.

52. Shellenbarger S. A crucial step for averting AI disasters. Wall St J 2019. Available at: https://www. wsj.com/articles/a-crucial-step-for-avoiding-ai-disasters-11550069865. Accessed May 9, 2021.

53. Abrams C. Google's effort to prevent blindness shows AI challenges. Wall Street J 2019. Available at: https://www.wsj.com/articles/googles-effort-to-prevent-blindness-hits-roadblock-11548504004. Accessed May 9, 2021.

54. Serchen J, Doherty R, Atiq O, et al. Racism and Health in the United States: A Policy Statement From the American College of Physicians. Ann Intern Med. 2020 Oct 6;173(7):556–7.

55. Diaz T, Navarro JR, Chen EH. An institutional approach to fostering inclusion and addressing racial bias: implications for diversity in academic medicine. Teach Learn Med 2020;32(1):110–6.

56. Osta K, Vazquez H. Implicit bias and structural racialization. Oakland, California: National Equity Project; 2020. Available at: https://www.nationalequityproject. org/frameworks/implicit-bias-structural-racialization#: %7E:text=Implicit%20bias%20(also%20referred% 20to,beliefs%20about%20fairness%20and% 20equality. Accessed July 31, 2020.

57. FitzGerald C, Hurst S. Implicit bias in healthcare professionals: a systematic review. BMC Med Ethics 2017;18(1):19.

58. Rajkomar A, Hardt M, Howell MD, et al. Ensuring fairness in machine learning to advance health equity. Ann Intern Med 2018;169(12):866–72.

59. Ford CL, Airhihenbuwa CO. Commentary: just what is critical race theory and what's it doing in a progressive field like public health? Ethn Dis 2018; 28(Suppl 1):223–30.

60. Eberly LA, Richterman A, Beckett AG, et al. Identification of Racial Inequities in Access to Specialized Inpatient Heart Failure Care at an Academic Medical Center. Circ Heart Fail 2019;12(11):e006214.

61. Morse M, Loscalzo J. Creating real change at academic medical centers - how social movements can be timely catalysts. N Engl J Med 2020;383(3): 199–201.

62. Lewsey SC, Breathett K. Racial and ethnic disparities in heart failure: current state and future directions. Curr Opin Cardiol 2021;36(3):320–8.

63. Johnson AE, Birru Talabi M, Bonifacino E, et al. Considerations for Racial Diversity in the Cardiology Workforce in the United States of America. J Am Coll Cardiol 2021;77(15):1934–7.

64. Currie G, Hawk KE. Ethical and legal challenges of artificial intelligence in nuclear medicine. Semin Nucl Med 2021;51(2):120–5.

65. Aggarwal N, Ahmed M, Basu S, et al. Advancing artificial intelligence in health settings outside the hospital and clinic. NAM Perspective. 2020. Available at: https://nam.edu/advancing-artificial-intelligence-in-health-settings-outside-the-hospital-and-clinic. Accessed June 10, 2021.

66. Barrett M, Boyne J, Brandts J, et al. Artificial intelligence supported patient self-care in chronic heart failure: a paradigm shift from reactive to predictive, preventive and personalised care. EPMA J 2019; 10(4):445–64.

67. Brewer LC, Fortuna KL, Jones C, et al. Back to the future: achieving health equity through health informatics and digital health. JMIR Mhealth and Uhealth 2020;8(1):e14512.

68. Noseworthy PA, Attia ZI, Brewer LC, et al. Assessing and mitigating bias in medical artificial intelligence: the effects of race and ethnicity on a deep learning Model for ECG Analysis. Circ Arrhythmia Electrophysiol 2020;13(3):e007988.

69. Wu X, Yuan X, Wang W, et al. Value of a machine learning approach for predicting clinical outcomes in young patients with hypertension. Hypertension 2020;75(5):1271–8.

70. Maragatham G, Devi S. LSTM model for prediction of heart failure in big data. J Med Syst 2019;43(5): 111.

71. Choi E, Schuetz A, Stewart WF, et al. Using recurrent neural network models for early detection of heart failure onset. J Am Med Inform Assoc 2017;24(2): 361–70.

72. Segar MW, Vaduganathan M, Patel KV, et al. Machine learning to predict the risk of incident heart failure hospitalization among patients with diabetes: The WATCH-DM Risk score. Diabetes care 2019; 42(12):2298–306.

73. Tabassian M, Sunderji I, Erdei T, et al. Diagnosis of heart failure with preserved ejection fraction: machine learning of spatiotemporal variations in left

ventricular deformation. J Am Soc Echocardiogr 2018;31(12):1272–84.e9.

74. Agliari E, Barra A, Barra OA, et al. Detecting cardiac pathologies via machine learning on heart-rate variability time series and related markers. Sci Rep 2020;10(1):8845.

75. Farmakis D, Koeck T, Mullen W, et al. Urine proteome analysis in heart failure with reduced ejection fraction complicated by chronic kidney disease: feasibility, and clinical and pathogenetic correlates. Eur J Heart Fail 2016;18(7):822–9.

76. Rossing K, Bosselmann HS, Gustafsson F, et al. Urinary Proteomics Pilot Study for biomarker discovery and diagnosis in heart failure with reduced ejection fraction. PLoS One 2016;11(6):e0157167.

77. Cho J, Lee B, Kwon JM, et al. Artificial Intelligence Algorithm for Screening Heart Failure with Reduced Ejection Fraction Using Electrocardiography. ASAIO J 2021;67(3):314–21.

78. Attia ZI, Kapa S, Yao X, et al. Prospective validation of a deep learning electrocardiogram algorithm for the detection of left ventricular systolic dysfunction. J Cardiovasc Electrophysiol 2019;30(5):668–74.

79. Zhang R, Ma S, Shanahan L, et al. Discovering and identifying New York heart association classification from electronic health records. BMC Med Inform Decis Mak 2018;18(Suppl 2):48.

80. Salem Omar AM, Shameer K, Narula S, et al. Artificial intelligence-based assessment of left ventricular filling pressures from 2-Dimensional cardiac ultrasound images. JACC Cardiovasc Imaging 2018;11(3):509–10.

81. Feeny AK, Rickard J, Patel D, et al. Machine learning prediction of response to cardiac resynchronization therapy: improvement versus current guidelines. Circ Arrhythmia Electrophysiol 2019;12(7):e007316.

82. Hirata Y, Kusunose K, Tsuji T, et al. Deep learning for detection of elevated pulmonary artery wedge pressure using standard chest X-Ray. Can J Cardiol. 2021 Aug;37(8):1198–206.

83. Hearn J, Ross HJ, Mueller B, et al. Neural networks for prognostication of patients with heart failure. Circ Heart Fail 2018;11(8):e005193.

84. Kwon JM, Kim KH, Jeon KH, et al. Deep learning for predicting in-hospital mortality among heart disease patients based on echocardiography. Echocardiography 2019;36(2):213–8.

85. Przewlocka-Kosmala M, Marwick TH, Dabrowski A, et al. Contribution of cardiovascular reserve to prognostic categories of heart failure with preserved ejection fraction: a classification based on machine learning. J Am Soc Echocardiogr 2019;32(5):604–15.e6.

86. Allam A, Nagy M, Thoma G, et al. Neural networks versus Logistic regression for 30daysall -causereadmission prediction. Sci Rep 2019;9(1):9277.

87. Tokodi M, Schwertner WR, Kovács A, et al. Machine learning-based mortality prediction of patients undergoing cardiac resynchronization therapy: the SEMMELWEIS-CRT score. Eur Heart J 2020;41(18):1747–56.

Using Artificial Intelligence to Better Predict and Develop Biomarkers

Sam A. Michelhaugh, BA[a,1], James L. Januzzi Jr, MD[b,c,d],*

KEYWORDS

- Genomics • Transcriptomics • Proteomics • Metabolomics • Artificial intelligence • Biomarkers
- Heart failure

KEY POINTS

- Biomarker discovery has been enhanced by the high-throughput technologies of omics.
- Artificial intelligence improves statistical analysis of the large data sets generated in omics to enhance identification of markers of potential interest.
- Application of omics, especially proteomics, has aided with identification of biomarkers with clinical relevance to heart failure.
- Through biomarker discovery, researchers can further study identified biomarkers to determine clinical utility, pathophysiology, and improve patient care.

INTRODUCTION

Given the complex pathophysiology and etiologies of heart failure (HF), tailoring care to improve patient outcomes and quality of life involves the integration of multiple parameters.[1] Beyond adjusting treatments based on symptoms and physical examination findings, clinicians must rely on adjunctive testing to support their judgment; this includes imaging and measurement of circulating biomarkers. Most notably, among biomarkers measured, natriuretic peptides are considered the standard of care for treating patients with HF.[2,3] However, HF is a complicated condition, which cannot be summarized by one biomarker alone.[4,5] Although natriuretic peptides indicate cardiomyocyte stretch, they have limited ability to capture other changes associated with HF remodeling included inflammation, oxidative stress, and fibrosis.[6,7] For this reason, multiple markers are needed to recognize the pathophysiology of HF and tailor care to optimize patient outcomes.

The introduction of omics, including genomics, transcriptomics, proteomics, and metabolomics, has enhanced biomarker discovery.[8–11] Omics allows for analysis of biological pathways involved in aspects of the central dogma and biological modifications of products. Using high-throughput and untargeted omics technologies provides better phenotyping and unveils previously unknown HF pathophysiology. Furthermore, integration of findings of multiple omics studies gives a comprehensive understanding of pathophysiology from the level of genes to final metabolites to recognize where disease processes arise.[12–14] Discovery of markers enables researchers and clinicians to recognize potential risks for developing HF, serve

a Georgetown University School of Medicine, Washington, DC, USA; b Department of Medicine, Division of Cardiology, Massachusetts General Hospital, 55 Fruit Street, Boston, MA 02114, USA; c Department of Medicine, Division of Cardiology, Harvard Medical School, Boston, MA, USA; d Baim Institute for Clinical Research, Boston, MA, USA
1 2500 Wisconsin Avenue Northwest, APT 948, Washington, DC 20007.
* Corresponding author.
E-mail address: jjanuzzi@partners.org

Heart Failure Clin 18 (2022) 275–285
https://doi.org/10.1016/j.hfc.2021.11.004
1551-7136/22/© 2021 Elsevier Inc. All rights reserved.

as prognostic indicators, or ascertain druggable targets for future therapeutic interventions.[15]

BACKGROUND

Previous work in biomarker research involved the testing of suspected markers individually. Through this process, individual markers were selected from proposed biological processes or previous research results. This hypothesis-driven process is inefficient and costly in terms of money, time, and sample used for each experiment.[16] With the advent of omics, experimenters can test multiple markers simultaneously.[12–14] Beyond improving throughput and decreasing waste, omics reduces bias as it is inductive, and allows for the identification of markers that may have otherwise not been considered.[17,18]

Modern omics technologies have great potential for researchers to improve efficiencies. In individual experiments, it is possible to test hundreds to thousands of individual targets simultaneously while using as little as 1 μL of sample or using a single cell.[19–21] Omics experiments are also being aided by technological advancements. Previous analysis would involve intensive statistics to sort through large data sets to identify markers of interest. Use of artificial intelligence (AI) in analysis makes result interpretation easier, faster, and more feasible for researchers who do not have access to biostatisticians capable of analyzing such data (**Fig. 1**).[12–14,22–24] We will discuss the broad range of omics possibilities but then focus on the area of proteomics.

THE OMICS MULTIVERSE
Genomics

In contrast to genetics (the study of heredity), genomics is the study of the entirety of all deoxyribonucleic acid (DNA) within an organism (**Fig. 2**). In certain diseases with underlying genetic components, understanding the genome helps identify patients at risk for developing particular diseases. With improved DNA sequencing technologies, the genome can be characterized through genome-wide association studies (GWASs). GWAS aims to identify variations in genes, such as single nucleotide polymorphisms, a substitution of an individual DNA base in the sequence.[12,13,25] Genomics in HF research has unveiled new insights into HF pathophysiology, such as identification of 2 loci where single nucleotide polymorphisms may predict future development of HF.[26–28]

Original DNA sequencing relied on the Sanger method, whereas newer and more efficient processes for conducting genomics have been developed. The Sanger method involves random fragmentation of single-stranded DNA samples, and replication using polymerase chain reaction. This involves combining samples with labeled dideoxynucleotide bases, primer, polymerase, and DNA bases. Replication of DNA strands will occur until random inclusion of a dideoxynucleotide base. The samples are then separated by size using gel electrophoresis and labeled dideoxynucleotide give information regarding terminal base and distance traveled gives size. Combining this information with the other fragments provides the DNA sequence.[25,29–31] Today other platforms such as DNA microarrays (discussed in the proteomics section) are used as they are higher throughput for identifying single nucleotide polymorphisms and are less prone to experimental error.[29,31]

Transcriptomics

Transcriptomics studies the ribonucleic acid (RNA) expressed by a cell both involved in coding proteins (mRNA, rRNA, and tRNA) and noncoding RNA (**Fig. 3**). Coding RNA gives insights into the proteins translated by the cell and noncoding shows possible posttranscriptional modulation of protein translation.[12,20] Other noncoding RNA, notably microRNA (RNA sequences between 18 and 25 nucleotides long) and long noncoding RNA (lncRNA, RNA sequences over 200 nucleotides long) are gaining interest as their role in regulating protein translation is being better understood.[20,32] Characterization of the dynamic transcriptome gives researchers upstream and downstream insight into HF pathologies such as identifying dysregulated genes in HF with preserved ejection fraction (HFpEF).[33] Given the similarity between DNA and RNA, modalities to sequence the genome can be applied to transcriptomics as well. This includes RNA-specific forms of microarrays and Sanger sequencing.[31,34]

Proteomics

Characterization of proteome provides insights into disease states and underlying pathophysiologies at the level of proteins (see **Fig. 3**). Beyond identifying potential biomarkers, proteomics can quantify proteins, determine regulation relative to normal or other timepoints, and determine posttranslational modifications such as phosphorylation.[35] Through AI, protein-protein interaction can be determined to elucidate pathophysiology and develop targeted therapies.[12,13,24,36]

Although protein biomarker discovery previously involved hypothesis generation and individual marker testing, modern methods are high

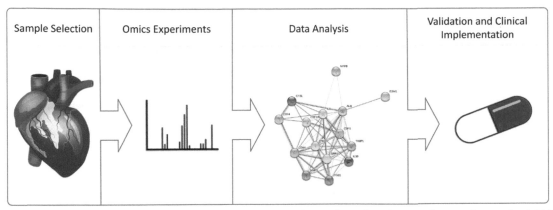

Fig. 1. Process of HF biomarker discovery. In discovering HF biomarkers, first the sample must be acquired. This can be either directly acquired cardiac tissue for measuring local markers, or blood sera or urine to measure circulating markers. The sample then undergoes genomics, transcriptomics, proteomics, or metabolomics either in isolation or using a combination of methods. Data are analyzed using artificial intelligence methods such as principal components analysis, random forest, and support vector machine models. After marker discovery, results can be validated with potential clinical utility as prognostic or diagnostic markers and druggable targets.

throughput with improved sensitivity and selectivity to detect low abundance proteins, and consume minimal sample.[19] The 4 most common modalities of proteomics are mass spectrometry (MS), protein microarrays, aptamer, and proximity extension assays (PEAs), which will be discussed in more detail in the *Approaches* section. These proteomic strategies improve knowledge of HF pathophysiology and can identify potential biomarkers of developing HF, HF diagnostic and prognostic biomarkers, and markers associated with HF prevention, and ultimately improve HF patient care.[8–11]

Metabolomics

The final major omics field is metabolomics, which studies the downstream, metabolic products of cellular processes (see **Fig. 3**). These include amino acids, carbohydrates, fatty acids, nucleic acids, and inorganic molecules.[12,13] In HF research, metabolomics can aid clinicians and researchers in understanding how certain pathologies use different metabolic processes.[37,38] For example, metabolic markers such as phosphatidylcholine and lysophosphatidylcholine (phospholipid metabolites), ornithine (an amino acid metabolite), isocitrate and hydroxybutyrate (cellular energy metabolites), and cotinine (a nicotine metabolite) were associated with an increased risk of developing HF in previously healthy individuals.[38]

Similar to proteomics, MS can characterize the metabolome in an unbiased manner.[12,13] In addition, nuclear magnetic resonance spectroscopy

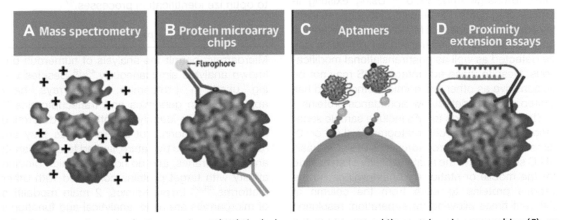

Fig. 2. Proteomic methods. Proteomic methods include mass spectrometry (*A*), protein microarray chips (*B*), aptamers (*C*), and proximity extension assays (*D*). Each method has its strengths and shortcomings, allowing for different utilities depending on the application. (*From* Michelhaugh SA, Januzzi JL. Finding a Needle in a Haystack: Proteomics in Heart Failure. *JACC Basic to Transl Sci.* 2020;5(10):1043-1053; with permission.)

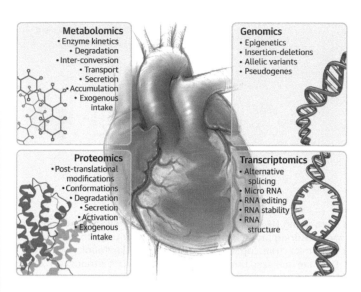

Fig. 3. Overview of omics fields and uses. Omics allows for characterization of the pathophysiology of heart failure in multiple dimensions. As heart failure is a multifaceted disease, a deeper understanding at the level of genes, transcripts, proteins, and metabolites is necessary. (*From* Michelhaugh SA, Januzzi JL. Finding a Needle in a Haystack: Proteomics in Heart Failure. *JACC Basic to Transl Sci.* 2020;5(10):1043-1053; with permission.)

can determine structures, and therein identities of analytes of separated samples using magnetic fields.[12,13,39,40] Likewise, Fourier Transformed Infrared Spectroscopy (FTIR) can identify unknown metabolites, although with less utility as FTIR can only provide information regarding functional groups. However, FTIR is nondestructive and can analyze solid, liquid, or gas samples.[39]

APPROACHES IN PROTEOMICS FOR IDENTIFICATION OF BIOMARKERS
MS Proteomics

MS is a powerful analytical technique for identifying unknown samples. Unlike other proteomic techniques, MS is destructive, as analyte is fragmented before being ionized and sorted by mass-to-charge (m/z) ratio.[41] Using existing libraries, fragments can be pieced together to identify analytes. A benefit of MS is it is untargeted and proteins across the characterized proteome can be detected as well as posttranslational modifications. Despite these advantages, MS may not be as sensitive as other proteomic methods and has limited ability to detect low-abundance proteins.

Standard methods for MS include sample separation using liquid chromatography (LC) or 2-dimensional gel electrophoresis (2-DE). The basis of LC separation is the relative affinity of an analyte for the mobile or stationary phase will cause the various proteins to elute from the column at different times allowing for separation; resolution can be improved by changing the polarity of the different phases.[41,42] In 2-DE, an unknown protein mixture is separated on a gel matrix first by pH until the protein reaches its isoelectric point (has no net charge), and then perpendicularly using electrophoresis to separate proteins by mass.[43,44] Although both methods can be fine-tuned to improve separation, LC is more common as it produces better resolution and is easily coupled to MS instruments.

After separation, samples must be ionized, usually using either matrix-assisted laser desorption ionization or electrospray ionization.[41,45] After ionization, the fragments must be separated by m/z ratio using either time of flight (TOF) or quadrupole analyzers. The m/z ratios of fragments findings can be compared to databases such as the National Institute of Standards and Technology.[46] Although identification of peptides from fragments was once a tedious process, machine learning has increased the ease of this process by generating algorithms to optimize identification processes.[47]

Protein Microarray Proteomics

Microarrays permit the analysis of numerous unknown analytes simultaneously.[48,49] Besides being used in proteomics, microarrays have applications in genomics and transcriptomics.[31] Microarrays can identify, quantify, and determine protein interactions, but are limited as they are relatively targeted by nature, limited to established antibody libraries, and do not have a high binding affinity with target proteins compared with other platforms.[48,49] In proteomics, 2 main modalities of microarrays are used: analytical and functional microarrays.

Analytical microarrays aim to identify and quantify proteins that are differentially regulated. Although there are several methods, the most common involves capture antibodies which have previously been determined to have binding affinity for target proteins are attached to a plate. Next, the sample is added to the plate and binding occurs if the antibody is specific for the protein. A reporter antibody with fluorescent or radioactive marker is then added and attaches to the capture antibody-protein complex. The complex can then be detected and quantified to provide information about the sample.[50] In functional microarrays, the identified proteins of interest are attached to the plate and are exposed to conditions such as drugs, lipids, DNA, and RNA to determine protein interactions.[49]

Aptamer Proteomics

Much like microarray proteomics, aptamer proteomics allows for testing numerous proteins simultaneously based on binding affinity to a previously characterized target. However, in this proteomics modality, short, tightly coiled oligonucleotide strands rather than antibodies are used. This difference creates more specific binding of aptamer to protein compared with protein microarrays.[51] Higher specificity is the result of aptamer design, and the complex sample processing, which has multiple steps to remove excess reagents and off-target binding products.[16,51,52]

Despite these successes, aptamer proteomics has its shortcomings. First, as it is relatively targeted because of the limited aptamer library, it has the potential of introducing bias in the analysis. The results generated from aptamer proteomics are relative concentrations, which cannot be compared to findings from other assays.[52] The sample processing involves multiple steps, introducing the possibility of human error.[51] The specificity of aptamer to protein introduces possible concerns. Although there is strong specificity for aptamers for target proteins, there is potential for cross-reactivity of different protein targets if the sequence and structure are conserved at the aptamer binding site.[10] The high affinity binding may not occur if there are posttranslational modifications.

PEA Proteomics

PEA is a proteomics method with great promise in biomarker discovery. Like microarrays, PEA involves binding of 2 antibodies to proteins in the sample. Instead of using radioactive or fluorescent markers, the protein-binding antibodies contain complimentary, short, single-stranded oligonucleotide sequences on the F_c region. The antibodies are designed so the F_{ab} portions bind the target protein in proximity such that the oligonucleotides

will hybridize. The hybridized oligonucleotide can be amplified using quantitative polymerase chain reaction.[53,54]

Advantages of PEA over other proteomics platforms is high sensitivity, reduced cross-reactivity, and ability to detect low concentrations of proteins. PEA only requires 1 µL of sample, making it beneficial when conserving sample for other analyses.[19] Limitations of PEA are inability to detect posttranslational modifications, bias introduced by targeted approach, and currently limited library.[55,56]

STATISTICAL ANALYSIS OF OMICS DATA

In the past, large and complicated data sets generated by omics required extensive statistical analysis. However, increased access to AI has improved analysis of omics data sets. Although there are several methods to analyze omics, the major methods include principal components analysis (PCA), random forest models, and support vector machines (SVMs) (**Table 1**).

PCA allows for related groups of proteins, referred to as features, to be extracted using orthogonal (90°) or oblique (<90°) rotations. Orthogonal rotations have been widely used in HF proteomic research because of the relative ease of analysis. However, this does not depict the one-to-many relationships proteins have in biological systems.[57] Once feature extraction is complete, individual proteins of interest are identified using matrixes.[58]

Random forest models use a series of decision trees to classify data based on supervised teaching data. To construct the random forest, numerous decision trees are created using different variables as the initial nodes and selecting a random number of variables at each step of the tree. From there, a bootstrap aggregate data set is used with the different trees and categorized. Using a system of majority voting where the greatest number of categorizations for one data point, the final classification is determined.[59,60]

SVMs are another form of supervised machine learning used in biomarker discovery analysis. Using training data sets of known classifications, groups are separated using a hyperplane (a line if there are 2 input features and a plane if there are 3 input features). Although many hyperplanes may correctly separate the data, the hyperplane that results in the greatest distance from the points in each cluster closest to the hyperplane, known as the margin, is chosen. Large margins will aid with classification of data that may otherwise not

Table 1
Comparison of omics analysis methods

Method	Strengths	Weaknesses
Principal components analysis	• Reduces overfitting • Reduces noise in data	• Use of oblique rotations is computationally more difficult • Unsupervised learning
Random forest model	• Reduces overfitting • Supervised learning	• Computationally complex • Training period is longer than other methods
Support vector machine	• Supervised learning • Not influenced by outliers	• Prone to overfitting • Does not explain data as well as other methods • Not as effective when datapoints overlap

be as discernible with smaller margins; however, this process may result in overfitting.[8,61]

The function, structure, and interactions of proteins identified can be better understood using AI and established databases. Gene ontology terms define proteins' functions to aid understanding pathophysiology of identified markers. Likewise, the Kyoto Encyclopedia of Genes and Genome provides pathway analysis to shed light on the role of identified proteins in disease mechanisms.[58] Other tools such as the Search Tool for the Retrieval of Interacting Genes/Proteins demonstrates protein-protein interactions.[62] Motif analysis can help gain insight to protein sequence, structure, and posttranslational modifications that may be associated with specific pathologies.[58]

AI has made *in silico* biomarker prediction possible. Although it is not currently used extensively in HF research, other fields have used data sets from several large proteomic studies to generate panels of proteins associated with various cancers[63] and Alzheimer's disease.[64] In hepatocellular carcinoma research, neural networks, a subdivision of machine learning, was used to identify prognostic markers.[65] Although predicted markers will require further validation, AI can economically identify potential biomarkers and conserves samples for biomarker validation.

METHODOLOGIC CONSIDERATIONS

When designing biomarker discovery experiments, there are several considerations. One decision is sample source. Although most proteomics studies test serum, it may be difficult to detect proteins with low expression.[16,52] Other sample types, such as tissue, provide insights to the local proteome within the heart but are difficult to obtain.[66] Urine samples, although easily obtained are not without their shortcomings. Proteins in

urine and are more representative of immediate processes and thus is more susceptible to minute-to-minute changes. The urine proteome requires characterization before becoming readily used.[67–69]

After determining sample type, the proteomics modality must be decided. Important considerations include choosing between an untargeted method such as MS (which is better suited for broad marker discovery) or targeted methods such as PEA (which as better suited for validation of previous findings and quantification).[13,70] Some techniques are better suited for certain applications, like using MS if there are concerns of posttranslational modifications affecting binding to aptamers.[71] Proteins involved in specific pathologies may have cross-reactivity, affecting results.[10] Even within a method, other parameters should be adjusted, including separation techniques in MS, and selection of protein panels in PEA, for example.

The final considerations are related to analysis of omics data. When deciding whether to use a targeted versus untargeted approach, targeted methods inherently introduce selection bias.[13,14,17,70,72] Other statistical alterations, such as changing false discovery rates and significance thresholds, for example, have the potential to greatly change data interpretation and results.[57,72] Care must be taken to ensure considerations align with the aims of the interpretation.

EXAMPLES OF STUDIES

The application of proteomics in HF research has uncovered new insights into disease processes. The following studies demonstrate how proteomics of various platforms can be used to discover biomarkers to aid in identifying those at risk for developing HF, predicting disease progression, and understanding mechanism of disease progression and treatments.

MS Proteomics of Urine Samples

Although many studies have applied MS proteomics to discover biomarkers associated with HF with reduced ejection fraction (HFrEF) using blood samples, Rossing and colleagues used urine samples from 127 patients with HFrEF, 581 controls without HF, and 176 with left ventricular diastolic dysfunction (LVDD) to discover potential markers of HFrEF and LVDD.[8] In their experimental design, spontaneous urine samples underwent capillary electrophoresis separation coupled MS using electrospray ionization and TOF analyzer.[8]

In an initial discovery phase, Rossing and colleagues analyzed the proteome of 33 HFrEF patients and 29 age-matched and sex-matched control patients without HF, ultimately identifying 103 peptides associated with HF. These peptides were predominately associated with the extracellular matrix (collagen type I and III and alpha-1-antitrypsin). After identifying peptides, machine learning was used to develop a system of weighting the amplitudes of MS peaks; the model generated was applied to 94 additional HFrEF patients to validate with 93.6% sensitivity, 92.9% specificity, and an area under the curve (AUC) of 0.972 (0.957–0.984, $P < .0001$). Interestingly, among 20 patients with preclinical HFrEF, the model had a sensitivity of 95%.[8]

Protein Microarray Proteomics to Discover Diagnostic and Prognostic Markers

Although not as commonly used as other modalities of proteomics and biomarker discovery, protein microarrays can successfully detect low quantities of proteins.[9] Jiang and colleagues used this platform to gain further insights into HFpEF. Currently, there are fewer markers for diagnosis and prognosis of HFpEF, which negatively impacts care for this patient population. In a small pilot sample of 3 HFpEF patients (defined as having New York Heart Association [NYHA] class III or IV HF, a left ventricular ejection fraction [LVEF] of greater than 40%, and N-terminal B-type natriuretic peptide [NT-proBNP] greater than 1500 pg/mL), 3 hypertensive patients, and 3 healthy control patients, sera samples underwent microarray testing. In their analysis, 507 proteins were tested and ultimately identified 59 significantly upregulated proteins, 11 of which were expressed more than 5-fold greater in HFpEF patients relative to control; 17 proteins were significantly upregulated in HFpEF relative to the hypertensive group and 1 was upregulated 5 times greater. Common

to both analyses of being upregulated greater than 5 times to its comparison group was angiogenin.[9]

Angiogenin is a marker of angiogenesis and has previously been thought to be involved in HF pathophysiology.[9,73] After identification of this potential HFpEF biomarker, Jiang and colleagues performed angiogenin immunohistochemistry validation in 16 HFpEF patients (LVEF = 41-49%, n = 9; LVEF $\geq$ 50%, n = 7) and 16 healthy controls. After adjusting for risk factors including age, sex, hypertension, and diabetes, angiogenin was elevated in both HFpEF groups relative to control. However, there was no statistical difference between the 2 ejection fraction cutoffs. When angiogenin was used as a predictor of HFpEF, it was found that the AUC was 0.88 (95% confidence interval, 0.73–1.00; $P < .001$), with a sensitivity of 81% and specificity of 94%. Despite the diagnostic and prognostic power of angiogenin, it did not serve as a predictor of all-cause death at 36-month follow-up.[9]

Aptamer Proteomics to Predict Incident Heart Failure

Prediction of HF using biomarkers is beneficial to clinicians as it allows for more aggressive and targeted interventions to prevent progression. Although markers like NT-proBNP have previously been identified as having predictive value for developing HF, additional markers are needed to better predict progression.[74] Nayor and colleagues aimed to identify protein biomarkers associated with cardiac remodeling as evidenced through echocardiographic parameters using aptamer-based proteomics. In their setup, the investigators included 1895 patients from the Framingham Heart Study without HF at baseline and measured up to 1305 proteins. Protein levels were then compared to various echocardiographic measures; it was ultimately found that 17 proteins were differentially regulated with regards to echocardiographic measures of left ventricular (LV) mass, LV diastolic dimension, and left atrial diameter.[10]

In another prospective analysis, the proteome of 174 patients who developed incident HF from baseline was compared to 1711 individuals who remained HF-free. From this examination, 29 proteins were associated with incident HF. When comparing these 29 potential biomarkers, no statistical difference was observed between those who developed HFpEF and HFrEF. When repeated using samples from the Nord-Trøndelag Health Study (n = 2497), a meta-analysis of the 149 patients with incident HF and 174 from the

Framingham Heart Study yielded 6 differentially regulated proteins. Three of these proteins were upregulated (NT-proBNP, thrombospondin-2, and mannose-binding lectin) and 3 were downregulated (epidermal growth factor receptor, growth differentiation factor 8/11, and hemojuvelin).[10]

Nayor and colleagues identified proteins associated with HF development measured with a mean of 19 years before follow-up in the Framingham Heart Study cohort. This suggests possible prediction of incident HF and identification of at-risk patients after further validation.

PEA to Identify Potential Targets to Prevent or Treat Heart Failure

Identifying specific interventions to prevent the development of HF remains a goal of HF clinicians. Although some treatments prevent progression to HF, notably β-blockers, angiotensin receptor blockers, and angiotensin-converting enzyme inhibitors, gaining a better mechanistic understanding of how these therapies prevent HF development will allow for more targeted therapeutic interventions in the future.[11,75] Using PEA proteomics, Ferreira and colleagues hoped to describe the mechanism of how spironolactone, a mineralocorticoid receptor antagonist, is able to improve survival in HF patients and prevent HF development.

In a randomized trial of adults aged 65 years or older receiving spironolactone (n = 265) or standard of care (n = 262), targeted PEA was performed on samples collected from baseline and follow-up at 1 and 9 months after enrollment to measure 276 proteins. Relative to control, those receiving spironolactone significantly downregulated 18 proteins and upregulated 33 proteins between baseline and 9 months after enrollment. When also examining changes between baseline, 1-, and 9-month follow-up samples, 5 proteins were significantly downregulated and 14 were significantly upregulated. Using network analysis, the 10 most differentially regulated proteins were assigned to 3 different clusters of 6 biologic functions (adipocytokine signaling, renin-angiotensin-aldosterone pathway, extracellular matrix metabolism, insulin growth factor signaling, hemostasis, and immune response).[11]

These different functional groupings reflect the possible effect of spironolactone on remodeling processes involved in HF such as decreasing collagen synthesis, inflammation, and angiogenesis. Better characterization and directed therapeutic interventions may prevent progression of patients at risk from developing HF.[11]

In another study, PEA was used to evaluate changes in the proteome of individuals with HFrEF before and after initiation of angiotensin receptor/neprilysin inhibitor (ARNI) in those with moderately advanced HF and following unloading with left ventricular assist device (LVAD) placement among those with advanced HF. In this analysis, Michelhaugh and colleagues found 5 proteins (NT-proBNP, endothelial cell-specific molecule-1, cathepsin L1, osteopontin, and MCSF-1) were differentially regulated after treatment with ARNI and LVAD. This core protein signature for HF may serve as a more accurate diagnostic cluster for the diagnosis, serve as druggable targets, have prognostic utility, or be used to monitor HF care.[76]

SUMMARY

Advancements in omics and AI have improved researcher's ability to discover HF biomarkers. Rather than relying on hypothesis-driven, individual marker testing, omics has opened the door to high-throughput analyses of genome, transcriptome, proteome, and metabolome to gain deeper understandings of pathophysiology in HF. With future validation studies, the characterized markers can be developed into panels to predict and monitor HF in the clinic. Discovered markers can be used as targets to treat HF patients or design therapeutic interventions to prevent HF from developing in at-risk patients. As AI and omics technologies continue to evolve, the clinical utility will increase substantially, improving patient outcomes.

CLINICS CARE POINTS

- Greater accessibility to AI allows clinical researchers to expand biomarker prediction and discovery.

- Although powerful at discovering potential markers, further validation is required before implementing at the bedside.

- AI can potentially predict biomarkers associated with HF using previously measured omics data.

- Integration of multiple biomarkers increases understanding of heart failure pathophysiology, and clinically can aid in improving detection, treatments, and quality of life.

DISCLOSURE

Dr J.L. Januzzi is supported in part by the Hutter Family Professorship; has been a trustee of the American College of Cardiology; has received grant support from Novartis Pharmaceuticals and Abbott Diagnostics; has received consulting income from Abbott, Janssen, Novartis, and Roche Diagnostics; has participated in clinical endpoint committees/data safety monitoring boards for Abbott, AbbVie, Amgen, CVRx, Janssen, MyoKardia, and Takeda. Mr S.A. Michelhaugh has no relationships to disclose.

REFERENCES

1. Yancy CW, Jessup M, Chair V, et al. Practice Guideline 2013 ACCF/AHA Guideline for the Management of Heart Failure. J Am Coll Cardiol. 2013 Oct 15; 62(16):e147–239.

2. Troughton RW, Frampton CM, Yandle TG, et al. Treatment of heart failure guided by plasma amino-terminal brain natriuretic peptide (N-BNP) concentrations. Lancet 2000;355(9210):1126–30.

3. Troughton R, Felker GM, Januzzi JL. Natriuretic peptide-guided heart failure management. doi: 10.1093/eurheartj/eht463

4. Giannessi D. Multimarker approach for heart failure management: Perspectives and limitations. Pharma Res 2011;64(1):11–24.

5. Pemberton CJ, Ikeda Y, De Rosa S, et al. The Diagnostic and Therapeutic Value of Multimarker Analysis in Heart Failure. An Approach to Biomarker-Targeted Therapy. Front Cardiovasc Med 2020;7: 579567. www.frontiersin.org.

6. Burchfield JS, Xie M, Hill JA. Pathological ventricular remodeling: Mechanisms: Part 1 of 2. Circulation 2013;128(4):388–400.

7. Holzhauser L, Kim G, Sayer G, et al. The Effect of Left Ventricular Assist Device Therapy on Cardiac Biomarkers: Implications for the Identification of Myocardial Recovery. Curr Heart Fail Rep. 2018 Aug;15(4):250–259.

8. Rossing K, Bosselmann HS, Gustafsson F, et al. Urinary proteomics pilot study for biomarker discovery and diagnosis in heart failure with reduced ejection fraction. PLoS One 2016;11(6):e0157167.

9. Jiang H, Zhang L, Yu Y, et al. A pilot study of angiogenin in heart failure with preserved ejection fraction: a novel potential biomarker for diagnosis and prognosis? J Cell Mol Med. 2014 Nov;18(11): 2189–97.

10. Nayor M, Short MI, Rasheed H, et al. Aptamer-Based Proteomic Platform Identifies Novel Protein Predictors of Incident Heart Failure and Echocardiographic Traits. Circ Hear Fail 2020;13(5). https://doi.org/10.1161/CIRCHEARTFAILURE.119.006749.

11. Ferreira JP, Verdonschot J, Wang P, et al. Proteomic and Mechanical Analysis of Spironolactone in Patients at Risk for HF. JACC Hear Fail 2021;9(4): 268–77.

12. Hasin Y, Seldin M, Lusis A. Multi-omics approaches to disease. Genome Biol. 2017 May 5;18(1):8.

13. Vailati-Riboni M, Palombo V, Loor JJ. What are omics sciences?. In: Periparturient diseases of Dairy Cows: a systems Biology approach. Springer International Publishing; 2017. p. 1–7. https://doi.org/10.1007/978-3-319-43033-1_1.

14. Subramanian I, Verma S, Kumar S, et al. Multi-omics Data Integration, Interpretation, and Its Application. Bioinform Biol Insights 2020;14. https://doi.org/10.1177/1177932219899051.

15. Ahmad T, Fiuzat M, Pencina MJ, et al. Charting a Roadmap for Heart Failure Biomarker Studies NIH Public Access. JACC Hear Fail 2014;2(5):477–88.

16. Brody EN, Gold L, Lawn RM, et al. High-content affinity-based proteomics: Unlocking protein biomarker discovery. Expert Rev Mol Diagn 2010; 10(8):1013–22.

17. Zheng Y. Study Design Considerations for Cancer Biomarker Discoveries. J Appl Lab Med 2018;3(2): 282–9.

18. McDermott JE, Wang J, Mitchell H, et al. Challenges in biomarker discovery: Combining expert insights with statistical analysis of complex omics data. Expert Opin Med Diagn 2013;7(1):37–51.

19. Smith JG, Gerszten RE. Emerging affinity-based proteomic technologies for large-scale plasma profiling in cardiovascular disease. Circulation 2017;135(17):1651–64.

20. Chambers DC, Carew AM, Lukowski SW, et al. Transcriptomics and single-cell RNA-sequencing. Respirology 2019;24(1):29–36.

21. Kulkarni A, Anderson AG, Merullo DP, et al. Beyond bulk: A review of single cell transcriptomics methodologies and applications Graphical abstract HHS Public Access Author manuscript. Curr Opin Biotechnol 2019;58:129–36.

22. Lancellotti C, Cancian P, Savevski V, et al. Artificial Intelligence & Tissue Biomarkers: Advantages, Risks and Perspectives for Pathology. 2021. Cells. 2021 Apr 2;10(4):787.

23. D'adamo GL, Widdop JT, Giles EM, et al. The future is now? Clinical and translational aspects of "Omics" technologies. Immunol Cell Biol 2021;99:168–76.

24. Chen C, Hou J, Tanner JJ, et al. Molecular Sciences Bioinformatics Methods for Mass Spectrometry-Based Proteomics Data Analysis. Int J Mol Sci. 2020 Apr 20;21(8):2873.

25. Del Giacco L, Cattaneo C. Introduction to genomics. Methods Mol Biol 2012;823:79–88.

26. Smith NL, Felix JF, Morrison AC, et al. Association of genome-wide variation with the risk of incident heart failure in adults of European and African ancestry : A

prospective meta-analysis from the cohorts for heart and aging research in genomic epidemiology (CHARGE) consortium. Circ Cardiovasc Genet 2010;3(3):256–66.

27. Reza N, Owens AT. Advances in the Genetics and Genomics of Heart Failure. Curr Cardiol Rep 2020;22(11). https://doi.org/10.1007/s11886-020-01385-z.

28. Tayal U, Prasad S, Cook SA. Genetics and genomics of dilated cardiomyopathy and systolic heart failure. Genome Med 2017;9(1). https://doi.org/10.1186/s13073-017-0410-8.

29. Wright J. A primer on DNA sequencing for the practicing urologist. Urol Times Urol Cancer Care 2021;10(2). Available at: https://www.urologytimes.com/view/a-primer-on-dna-sequencing-for-the-practicing-urologist.

30. Shendure J, Balasubramanian S, Church GM, et al. DNA sequencing at 40: Past, present and future. Nature 2017;550(7676):345–53.

31. Gasperskaja E, Kučinskas V. The most common technologies and tools for functional genome analysis. Acta Med Litu 2017;24(1):1–11.

32. Fang Y, Fullwood MJ. Roles, Functions, and Mechanisms of Long Non-coding RNAs in Cancer. Genomics Proteomics Bioinformatics 2016;14(1):42–54.

33. Das S, Frisk C, Eriksson MJ, et al. Transcriptomics of cardiac biopsies reveals differences in patients with or without diagnostic parameters for heart failure with preserved ejection fraction. Sci Rep. 2019 Feb 28;9(1):3179.

34. Valdés A, Ibáñez C, Simó C, et al. Recent transcriptomics advances and emerging applications in food science. Trac - Trends Anal Chem 2013;52:142–54.

35. Mann M, Jensen ON. Proteomic analysis of post-translational modifications. Nat Biotechnol 2003;21(3):255–61.

36. Michelhaugh SA, Januzzi JL. Finding a Needle in a Haystack: Proteomics in Heart Failure. JACC Basic Transl Sci 2020;5(10):1043–53.

37. Tahir UA, Katz DH, Zhao T, et al. Metabolomic profiles and heart failure risk in black adults: Insights from the jackson heart study. Circ Heart Fail. 2021 Jan;14(1):e007275.

38. Andersson C, Liu C, Cheng S, et al. Metabolomic signatures of cardiac remodelling and heart failure risk in the community. ESC Hear Fail 2020;7(6):3707–15.

39. Bujak R, Struck-Lewicka W, Markuszewski MJ, et al. Metabolomics for laboratory diagnostics. J Pharm Biomed Anal 2015;113:108–20.

40. Kordalewska M, Markuszewski MJ. Metabolomics in cardiovascular diseases. J Pharm Biomed Anal 2015;113:121–36.

41. Timp W, Timp G. Beyond mass spectrometry, the next step in proteomics. Sci Adv 2020;6(2):eaax8978.

42. Ali I, Aboul-Enein HY, Singh P, et al. Separation of biological proteins by liquid chromatography. Saudi Pharm J 2010;18(2):59–73.

43. Ning F, Wu X, Wang W. Expert Review of Proteomics Exploiting the potential of 2DE in proteomics analyses Exploiting the potential of 2DE in proteomics analyses. Expert Rev Proteomics. 2016 Oct;13(10):901–3.

44. Lohnes K, Quebbemann NR, Liu K, et al. Combining high-throughput MALDI-TOF mass spectrometry and isoelectric focusing gel electrophoresis for virtual 2D gel-based proteomics. Methods 2016;104:163–9.

45. Aebersold R, Mann M. Mass spectrometry-based proteomics. Nature 2003;422(6928):198–207.

46. Stein S. Mass spectral reference libraries: An ever-expanding resource for chemical identification. Anal Chem 2012;84(17):7274–82.

47. Liebal UW, Phan ANT, Sudhakar M, et al. Machine learning applications for mass spectrometry-based metabolomics. Metabolites 2020;10(6):1–23.

48. Zhu H, Qian J. Applications of Functional Protein Microarrays in Basic and Clinical Research. Advances in genetics, 79. Academic Press Inc.; 2012. p. 123–55. https://doi.org/10.1016/B978-0-12-394395-8.00004-9.

49. Hu S, Xie Z, Qian J, et al. Functional Protein Microarray Technology. Wiley Interdiscip Rev Syst Biol Med 2011;3(3):255–68.

50. Macbeath G. Protein microarrays and proteomics. Nat Genet 2002;32(4S):526–32.

51. Gold L, Ayers D, Bertino J, et al. Aptamer-based multiplexed proteomic technology for biomarker discovery. PLoS One 2010;5(12). https://doi.org/10.1371/journal.pone.0015004.

52. Lollo B, Steele F, Gold L. Beyond antibodies: New affinity reagents to unlock the proteome. Proteomics 2014;14(6):638–44.

53. Assarsson E, Lundberg M, Holmquist G, et al. Homogenous 96-plex PEA immunoassay exhibiting high sensitivity, specificity, and excellent scalability. PLoS One 2014;9(4):e95192.

54. Lundberg M, Eriksson A, Tran B, et al. Homogeneous antibody-based proximity extension assays provide sensitive and specific detection of low-abundant proteins in human blood. Nucleic Acids Res. 2011 Aug;39(15):e102.

55. Solier C, Langen H. Antibody-based proteomics and biomarker research-current status and limitations. Proteomics 2014;14(6):774–83.

56. Graumann J, Finkernagel F, Reinartz S, et al. Multiplatform Affinity Proteomics Identify Proteins Linked to Metastasis and Immune Suppression in Ovarian Cancer Plasma. Front Oncol 2019;9:1150.

57. Lualdi M, Fasano M. Statistical analysis of proteomics data: A review on feature selection. J Proteomics 2019;198:18–26.

58. Schmidt A, Forne I, Imhof A. Bioinformatic analysis of proteomics data. BMC Syst Biol 2014;8(Suppl 2):S3.

59. Yang L, Wu H, Jin X, et al. Study of cardiovascular disease prediction model based on random forest in eastern China. Sci Rep 2020;10(1). https://doi.org/10.1038/S41598-020-62133-5.

60. Breiman L. Random Forests. Mach Learn 45, 5–32 (2001).

61. Cortes C. Support-Vector Networks. Mach Learn 20, 273–297 (1995).

62. Szklarczyk D, Gable AL, Lyon D, et al. STRING v11: Protein-protein association networks with increased coverage, supporting functional discovery in genome-wide experimental datasets. Nucleic Acids Res 2019;47(D1):D607–13.

63. Björling E, Lindskog C, Oksvold P, et al. A web-based tool for in silico biomarker discovery based on tissue-specific protein profiles in normal and cancer tissues. Mol Cell Proteomics 2008;7(5):825–44.

64. Greco I, Day N, Riddoch-Contreras J, et al. Alzheimer's disease biomarker discovery using in silico literature mining and clinical validation. J Transl Med 2012;10(1):1–10.

65. Chaudhary K, Poirion OB, Lu L, et al. Deep Learning based multi-omics integration robustly predicts survival in liver cancer. Clin Cancer Res 2018;24(6):1248.

66. Lam MPY, Ping P, Murphy E. Proteomics Research in Cardiovascular Medicine and Biomarker Discovery. J Am Coll Cardiol 2016;68(25):2819–30.

67. Gao YH. Urine-an untapped goldmine for biomarker discovery? Sci China Life Sci 2013;56(12):1145–6.

68. Jing J, Gao Y. Urine Biomarkers in the Early Stages of Diseases: Current Status and Perspective - Jian Jing - Discovery Medicine. Discov Med 2018; 25(136):57–65. Available at: https://www.discoverymedicine.com/Jian-Jing-2/2018/02/urine-biomarkers-in-the-early-stages-of-diseases-current-status-and-perspective/.

69. Gao Y. Urine is a better biomarker source than blood especially for kidney diseases. Adv Exp Med Biol 2015;845:3–12.

70. Sobsey CA, Ibrahim S, Richard VR, et al. Targeted and Untargeted Proteomics Approaches in Biomarker Development. Proteomics 2020;20(9). https://doi.org/10.1002/pmic.201900029.

71. Betzen C, Alhamdani MSS, Lueong S, et al. Clinical proteomics: Promises, challenges and limitations of affinity arrays. Proteomics - Clin Appl 2015;9(3–4):342–7.

72. Lay JO, Borgmann S, Liyanage R, et al. Problems with the '"omics. "' Trends Anal Chem 2006;25(11):1046–56.

73. Tello-Montoliu A, Patel JV. Lip GYH. Angiogenin: A review of the pathophysiology and potential clinical applications. J Thromb Haemost 2006;4(9):1864–74.

74. Campbell DJ, Gong FF, Jelinek MV, et al. Prediction of incident heart failure by serum amino-terminal pro-B-type natriuretic peptide level in a community-based cohort. Eur J Heart Fail 2019; 21(4):449–59.

75. Horwich TB, Fonarow GC. Prevention of heart failure. JAMA Cardiol 2017;2(1):116.

76. Michelhaugh SA, Camacho A, Ibrahim NE, et al. Proteomic Signatures During Treatment in Different Stages of Heart Failure. Circ Hear Fail 2020. https://doi.org/10.1161/circheartfailure.119.006794.

Advances in Machine Learning Approaches to Heart Failure with Preserved Ejection Fraction

Faraz S. Ahmad, MD, MS[a,b,c,1], Yuan Luo, PhD[b,c,2],
Ramsey M. Wehbe, MD, MSAI[a,c,1], James D. Thomas, MD[a,c,1],
Sanjiv J. Shah, MD[a,c,d,*,1]

KEYWORDS

- Heart failure • Artificial intelligence • Machine learning • Deep learning
- Natural language processing

KEY POINTS

- Heart failure with preserved ejection fraction is a heterogenous, morbid condition with several unmet needs.
- Machine learning has the potential to guide precision medicine approaches for heart failure with preserved ejection fraction, such as identification of rare causes, subphenotyping, and increasing the efficiency of clinical trial enrollment.
- Understanding the strengths, limitations, and pitfalls of machine learning approaches is critical to realizing the potential of machine learning to impact the health of the patient with heart failure with preserved ejection fraction.

INTRODUCTION

Heart failure (HF) is a common condition with a profound impact on patients and the health care system. Heart failure with preserved ejection fraction (HFpEF) comprises nearly half of all cases of HF, affects more than 3 million US adults, and is underdiagnosed.[1] Multiple risk factors and conditions, such diabetes, hypertension, obesity, metabolic syndrome, and aging, contribute to inflammation and endothelial dysfunction and ultimately lead to the multiorgan, systemic syndrome of HFpEF in many patients.[2] Others can develop the syndrome of HFpEF for other reasons, including owing to genetic variants (eg, hypertrophic cardiomyopathy), infiltration of the myocardium (such as cardiac amyloidosis), or other toxic-metabolic myocardial insults. Regardless its cause, HFpEF remains a

[a] Division of Cardiology, Department of Medicine, Northwestern University Feinberg School of Medicine, Chicago, IL, USA; [b] Department of Preventive Medicine, Northwestern University Feinberg School of Medicine, Chicago, IL, USA; [c] Bluhm Cardiovascular Institute Center for Artificial Intelligence, Northwestern Medicine, Chicago, IL, USA; [d] Center for Deep Phenotyping and Precision Therapeutics, Institute for Augmented Intelligence in Medicine, Northwestern University Feinberg School of Medicine, 676 North St. Clair Street, Suite 730, Chicago, IL 60611, USA
[1] Present address: 676 North St. Clair Street, Suite 600, Chicago, IL 60611.
[2] Present address: Rubloff Building, 11th Floor, 750 North Lake Shore, Chicago, IL 60611.
* Corresponding author. Bluhm Cardiovascular Institute, Division of Cardiology, Department of Medicine, Center for Deep Phenotyping and Precision Therapeutics, Institute for Augmented Intelligence in Medicine, Northwestern University Feinberg School of Medicine, 676 North St. Clair Street, Suite 730, Chicago, IL 60611, USA.
E-mail address: sanjiv.shah@northwestern.edu
Twitter: @FarazA (F.S.A.); @yuanhypnosluo (Y.L.); @ramseywehbemd (R.M.W.); @jamesdthomasMD1 (J.D.T.); @HFpEF (S.J.S.)

Heart Failure Clin 18 (2022) 287–300
https://doi.org/10.1016/j.hfc.2021.12.002

highly morbid condition that negatively impacts quality of life, is marked by frequent hospitalizations and high mortality, and has few therapeutic options despite numerous clinical trials testing various medications and devices. Machine learning (ML) has the potential to improve diagnosis and treatment of patients with HFpEF, although its impact thus far has been limited.

ML, a domain that arose from the fields of statistics and computer science, focuses on teaching computers to learn from data, interpret it, and make predictions. It enables Internet search, speech recognition, image identification, and human-computer interactions by learning from large data sets.[3–5] ML is not a new field but has been gaining considerable attention within the health care and cardiovascular research communities over the past several years. The reasons for this trend are likely multifactorial, in part because of improved processing power and the availability of large data sets with a large number of variables (features).[6,7] Indeed, the inability to interpret the increasingly high density of data coming from diverse sources in the clinical setting is one of the key reasons ML may be uniquely poised to help clinicians and researchers avoid a loss of potentially valuable information that could improve clinical decision-making and patient care.

HFpEF is a prototypical cardiovascular condition that may benefit from ML because of its inherent heterogeneity, the need for improved classification, and the challenges in HFpEF diagnosis and treatment.[8] Here, the authors first briefly highlight several unmet needs within the HFpEF field that may benefit from ML approaches. Next, they provide an overview of key types of ML and concepts within the field. The authors describe several challenges and pitfalls of ML and provide a roadmap for the evaluation of ML studies. Finally, they discuss future directions of ML in HFpEF and the broader field of precision cardiovascular medicine.

THE UNMET NEED FOR BETTER APPROACHES TO HEART FAILURE DIAGNOSIS AND MANAGEMENT

HFpEF is a heterogenous condition with multiple pathways that lead to its development. Identifying less common causes of HFpEF, such as cardiac amyloidosis, hypertrophic cardiomyopathy, and cardiac sarcoidosis, can be challenging. Earlier diagnosis of cardiomyopathies with specific treatment options may lead to improved quality of life and survival. For example, cardiac amyloidosis is likely far more common than previously realized and may comprise up to 5% to 7% of HFpEF cases.[9,10] Prior studies have revealed the presence of early clinical clues of cardiac amyloidosis, including symptoms, laboratory abnormalities, and changes on echocardiograms and electrocardiograms (ECG).[11–13] Identifying early signs is essential given the emergence of novel therapies that can halt cardiac amyloidosis disease progression and improve prognosis.[14,15]

Most patients with HFpEF develop the condition in the setting of one of more risk factors and conditions, such as diabetes, hypertension, obesity, metabolic syndrome, sedentary lifestyle, chronic kidney disease, and ischemic heart disease. Numerous clinical trials in patients with HFpEF have failed to show a difference in their primary outcome.[2,16] This may be in part due to the heterogeneity of patients with HFpEF and the need for better subclassification. ML can be used to uncover patterns in diverse data and identify subgroups of patients with distinct pathophysiologic profiles and potential differential responses to therapy. ML approaches are designed to leverage the vast amounts of available data and account for higher-order interactions, multidimensionality, and nonlinear effects and may complement conventional statistical methods.[17] ML algorithms can be applied to either data from HFpEF observational cohorts for identifying novel subgroups or predictors of adverse outcomes or data from HFpEF clinical trial participants for hypothesis-generating, post hoc analyses to identify subgroups of patients with HF who benefited from the intervention. Although there is some debate about whether responder analyses are possible in clinical trials, it is possible that lack of that targeting may explain why numerous clinical trials in HFpEF have failed to show a difference in their primary outcome.

Identifying appropriate patients and enrolling in HF clinical trials have become increasingly challenging, particularly in the United States. Despite the high prevalence of HF, in North America and Western Europe the typical clinical trial enrollment rate is a dismal 1 to 2 patients per year per site in HF trials.[18] For example, in the TOPCAT (Treatment of Preserved Cardiac Function Heart Failure with an Aldosterone Antagonist) trial, which randomized HFpEF patients to spironolactone versus placebo, the average US enrollment rate was only 1.4 patients per site per year even though HFpEF is a leading cause of hospitalization in the United States. This problem could be addressed by better identification of eligible patients through applying ML to electronic health record (EHR) data.

A substantial amount of literature exists on risk prediction for hospitalization and mortality in patients with HFpEF. Although most risk models for patients with HFpEF were developed in cohorts with all types of HF, there are a few models developed specifically for patients with HFpEF (such as the I-PRESERVE Score and ARIC Score).[19] Most models have modest discrimination and calibration at best.[19] ML has the potential to lead to the development of either higher performing models using more diverse data sources (ie, EHR, imaging, ECG, sensors) or a more parsimonious set of variables that will facilitate deployment with EHR systems. For example, the MARKER-HF (Machine Learning Assessment of RisK and EaRly mortality in Heart Failure) risk model uses 8 laboratory variables to predict 90-day and 1-year mortality and with similar performance to other risk models that require more data, much of which are not readily available in the EHR.[20,21] Thus, ML has the potential to improve prediction for patients with HFpEF, although trials studying the implementation of these algorithms as part of routine care will be needed before wider adoption.

OVERVIEW OF MACHINE LEARNING TECHNIQUES

Artificial intelligence (AI) broadly refers to computer systems designed to perform tasks that usually require human intelligence (**Fig. 1**). ML enables AI computer systems through learning from data without explicit programming. ML algorithms can be broadly categorized, depending on the nature of the data that are used in the training process. *Supervised learning* algorithms (**Fig. 2**) are given labeled training data, so that each training

instance consists of features (eg, age, gender, blood pressure, left ventricular ejection fraction) and a label (eg, HF diagnosis, mortality, HF hospitalization), indicating the class to which the instance belongs.[4] The algorithms then learn to predict the outcome or label based on the aforementioned features, with the goal of making accurate predictions in new patients. *Unsupervised learning* algorithms (see **Fig. 2**) are given unlabeled data and aim to discover intrinsic patterns in the data (eg, subpopulations such as subphenotypes, or clusters). A hybrid of these 2 approaches is called *semisupervised learning*, which uses a combination of labeled and unlabeled data.[22] Semisupervised algorithms can be particularly useful in building predictive models when limited amounts of labeled data are available. Last, *reinforcement learning* is a form of ML that seeks to find an optimal set of sequential actions in a prespecified environment/domain to maximize a defined reward or goal.[23] Reinforcement learning, which has been used to successfully teach computers how to play and win games (by sequentially playing the game and learning from mistakes), can also be applied to the health care setting (eg, if the authors want to ask how the sequence and timing of interventions affect outcomes).

TYPES OF MACHINE LEARNING APPROACHES
Supervised Machine Learning

In supervised learning, algorithms are developed using labeled training data (see **Fig. 2**). This means

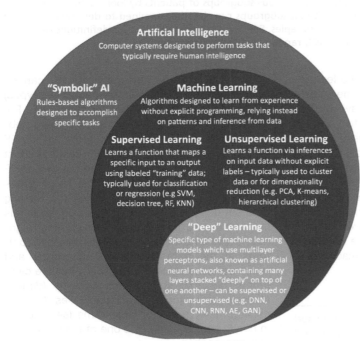

Fig. 1. AI and ML. The relationship between AI, ML, and "deep" learning. AE, autoencoder; CNN, convolutional neural network; DNN, deep neural network; GAN, generative adversarial network; KNN, k-nearest neighbor; PCA, principal components analysis; RF, random forests; RNN, recurrent neural network; SVM, support vector machines; VAE, variational autoencoder. (*From* Wehbe RM, Khan SS, Shah SJ, Ahmad FS. Predicting High-Risk Patients and High-Risk Outcomes in Heart Failure. Heart Fail Clin. 2020 Oct;16(4):387 to -407.)

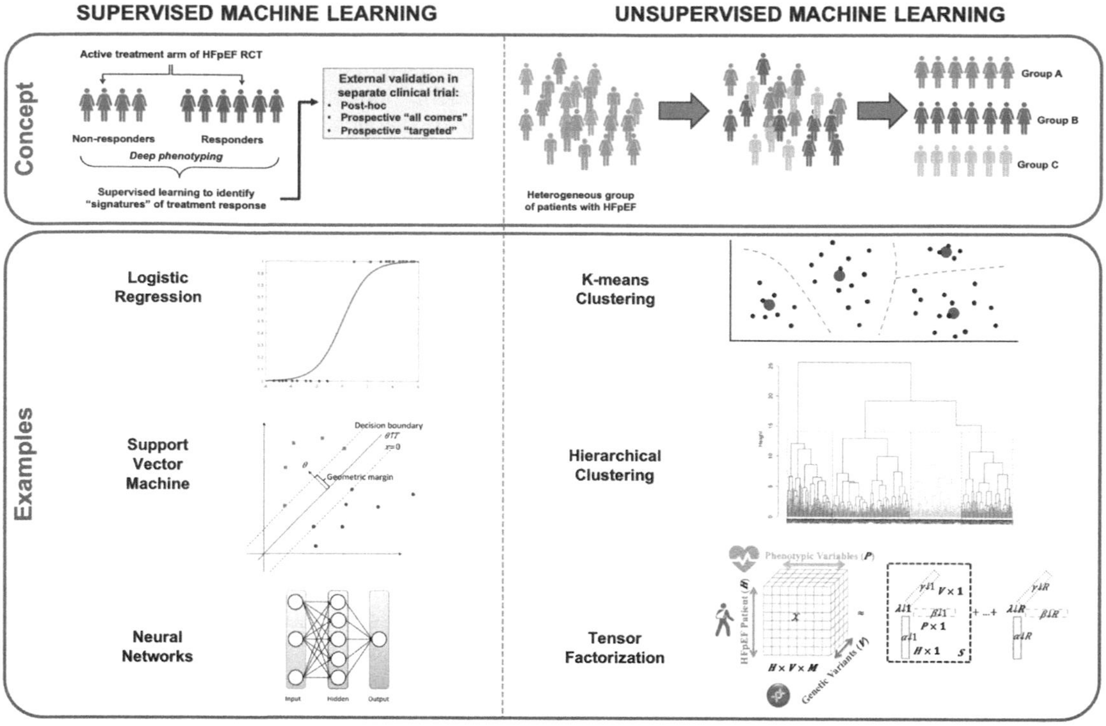

Fig. 2. Types of ML. In supervised ML, the outcomes (labels) are provided so that the ML algorithm can be trained to identify features that can successfully predict these outcomes (or labels) in external data sets. In the example provided, deep phenotypic data from the active treatment arm of an HFpEF clinical trial could be analyzed using a statistical learning approach in order to identify features ("signature") of treatment response. The resultant classifier could then be used to determine whether it could successfully predict treatment responders in a similar previously completed clinical trial (post hoc analysis) or in a new prospective trial of "all comers." Alternatively, patients could be screened by the classifier and only enrolled in a new, prospective, targeted treatment trial if they met criteria for being a "treatment responder." Unsupervised ML can be applied to a heterogeneous clinical syndrome, such as HFpEF, in order to identify homogeneous subgroups of patients by looking for intrinsic patterns within data from these patients. The identified subgroups can then be examined to determine whether they have differential outcomes or responses to therapies. See Supplementary Table 1 for definitions of the examples of ML algorithms shown in the figure. RCT, randomized controlled trial.

that for each item in the training set, the features (variables) are known, and the outcome is estimated. For example, several studies have attempted to use supervised ML to predict rehospitalization in HF patients. In these studies, the computer is told who was rehospitalized and who was not, and the algorithm may estimate for each participant whether he or she will be rehospitalized based on predefined features. There are several different supervised ML techniques, and each has its relative strengths and weaknesses. Examples of these approaches include linear and logistic regression, support vector machines,[24] and random forests.[25]

Unsupervised Machine Learning

Unsupervised learning differs from supervised learning in that the algorithms are developed based on intrinsic patterns in the data (ie, the data are unlabeled). Unsupervised ML can be used to identify subgroups (ie, subphenotypes) within a heterogeneous clinical syndrome. For example, suppose one wanted to identify subgroups within the clinical syndrome of HFpEF with the goal of designing a trial to test the effect of a targeted therapy on reducing the risk of HF hospitalization. They can cast this as an unsupervised learning problem in which the training data set does not come with preassigned labels (ie, "outcomes"). Unsupervised learning algorithms evaluate intrinsic relationships and patterns in the data to identify subgroups and reduce dimensionality and typically include clustering, principal components analysis (dimensionality reduction), association rules (pattern mining), or factorization algorithms (see **Fig. 2**). In health care, clustering is one of the most popular approaches.

Clustering creates groups of similar patients. Clustering algorithms have multiple variations, among which the most popular ones include k-means clustering, hierarchical clustering, and model-based clustering. The algorithms generally measure the distance between individual features to identify clusters, and there are several different methods for determining the optimal number of clusters.[26,27] Additional details on different types of clustering are included in Supplemental Table 1. Importantly, clustering is a way of dividing the population into groups so that patients are different across groups and similar within each group.

Beyond clustering, there are many other unsupervised learning techniques. For example, if there is a population of patients with HFpEF, one may expect a subgroup of patients to vary along 1 dimension (eg, general health status) that is reflected in many different aspects of their medical history (and thus many different features within the data set). In this case, dimensionality reduction methods like principal component analysis or factor analysis[28] are often used.

Deep Learning, Natural Language Processing, and Additional Machine Learning Techniques

Deep learning, which is an extension of neural networks, is a popular approach that attempts to overcome a major disadvantage of conventional ML techniques: their inability to effectively interpret and process high-dimensional raw signal data, such as audio and images.[5,29] As a result of this limitation, attempts to apply ML to echocardiographic data have mostly relied on measured and annotated quantitative measurements by highly experienced echocardiographers.[30] Instead, deep learning can often learn from raw data (such as the pixel values from an image or raw text from the EHR) using a hierarchy of increasingly complex and discriminative layers of processing. A key benefit of deep learning is its ability to learn features directly from data without the need for painstaking feature annotation by domain experts, a process known as feature *engineering*. Deep learning applications can have varying architectures, each with different strengths and limitations. These include convolutional neural networks, recurrent neural networks, autoencoders, and generative adversarial network.[5]

Deep learning is a technique that can be applied for very large data sets with either structured or unstructured data (eg, imaging or ECG repositories). Deep learning can also be applied to a smaller data set (eg, medical images), if there exists a similar large data set (eg, an archive of conventional photographic images) on which the analytical model can be pretrained in an approach called transfer learning.[31]

Natural language processing (NLP) applies computational algorithms to the problem of recovering structure from text and speech. These algorithms can be based on hand-coded rules, machine-learned models, or (commonly) a blend of both approaches. In the clinical domain, NLP can be used to extract clinically relevant information from a large number of clinical notes that are commonly found in the EHR.[32,33] In fact, deep learning algorithms have been applied with great success to many NLP tasks.[34] At the lowest level, NLP algorithms are used to segment text into words (or "tokens"), which can be further analyzed for parts of speech (eg, noun, verb, adjective), and other lexical features. Other NLP algorithms are then applied to recover higher-level linguistic structure, such as sentences, phrases, and sentential parses. These structures can subsequently be used as features for recognizing and extracting semantically meaningful chunks of information from text, such as entities that are mentioned and relations between these entities. In the clinical domain, such entities can be diseases, drugs, symptoms, and medications. They could also be events and their temporal properties, such as an adverse reaction occurring after treatment was performed or a drug prescribed.[35,36]

Transformers are a relatively novel class of deep learning methods for analyzing sequence data based on self-attention that have been leveraged with remarkable success for complex NLP tasks.[37] For example, researchers at Google (Mountain View, CA, USA)[38] developed Bidirectional Encoder Representations from Transformers (BERT), and multiple groups have extended this work by pretraining BERT models on corpuses of biomedical and clinical text and then testing those models on biomedical and health care tasks, including readmission prediction.[39–42] OpenAI (San Francisco, CA, USA), one of the leaders in developing generalized AI models, created the Generative Pre-trained Transformer 3,[43] which is a highly sophisticated language model that is able to generate text and conversations mimicking humans, although its adoption into health care settings will require additional research and thoughtful exploration of its potential and pitfalls.[44]

In the realm of clinical medicine, NLP can be an effective method to derive structured data from the EHR owing to the large amount of unstructured, free text entries in hospital and clinic notes, discharge summaries, imaging reports, procedure reports, and the like. In HFpEF, NLP can serve a variety of purposes, such as detecting HFpEF and cardiomyopathies, to assist with earlier diagnosis or providing data for use in developing strategies to reduce hospital readmissions in patients with HFpEF.[45–49] Leveraging NLP algorithms could have a significant impact on HFpEF clinical trials. For example, NLP-assisted identification of suitable clinical trial patients could save time and money, as it often takes study coordinators large amounts of time to screen single patients for HF trials, which often have complex inclusion and exclusion criteria. Applied in this manner, NLP could reduce the time needed for HF clinical trial screening from the EHR from several days (when done by humans) to just a few minutes when done by a computer.

When designing ML systems, the choice of the method, which depends on several factors, including the size of the data set, the number and informativeness of the features, and the ultimate research question or goal, is central.

Feature Selection, Hyperparameters, Overfitting, and Regularization

Feature selection is one of the most critical aspects of ML and depends on the task. For image classification, having large, labeled, and balanced data sets is key to successful model development. For other tasks, such as subtyping HFpEF with clinical data, selecting features that are informative and orthogonal increase the likelihood of identifying meaningful clusters.

Aside from feature selection, there are design choices that must be made by the ML scientist when training an ML model. These model parameters that are explicitly set to control the learning process are called "hyperparameters" (eg, model algorithm/architecture and size, learning rate, number of clusters in unsupervised learning). Theoretically, these hyperparameters could be tuned such that a given model would fit the training data perfectly. However, such a model would be unlikely to generalize well to new, unseen data sets because it would have modeled noise inherent in the training data set in addition to the true relationship between data inputs and outputs/labels. This is an example of *overfitting* and is a consequence of the concept of the *bias-variance tradeoff*.

A model that has overfit to training data but does not generalize well to external data sets would be said to have *low bias* and *high variance*; *bias* is an expression of the error of the model in approximating a complex function that governs real-life processes, whereas *variance* is an expression of the sensitivity of model performance to subtle changes from 1 data set to the next. Conversely, a model that is *underfit* is said to have *high bias*

and *low variance*, likely because it is too simplistic to approximate the true underlying relationship between data inputs and outputs. Such a model would perform poorly on the given task, but performance would be robust to subtle changes from 1 data set to the next. The goal in training any model is to attempt to resolve this tradeoff and minimize both bias and variance as much as possible.

There are several strategies to resolve this tradeoff on a given data set, including acquiring additional training data, adjusting the complexity of the model, and methods such as model ensembling, transfer learning, and regularization. Regularization refers to a family of methods that impose some sort of penalty or constraint on the model to prevent overly confident predictions and overfitting on the training data. Examples include penalized regression, data augmentation, dropout, and early stopping of the training process. The idea of regularization is foundational for most ML techniques.[50]

Train-Test Paradigm

During the training process, it is crucial that the ML scientist monitor for overfitting. This is done via a *validation data set*. Validation data sets can be a hold-out partition of the training set or alternatively when data size is limited can take the form of k-fold cross-validation, where the training set is iteratively partitioned into k number of subsets, with 1 subset being used as the validation data set during each iteration. It is important to note that this is distinct from the concept of "validation data sets" used to validate a given model in the risk prediction literature. In contrast, validation data sets in ML are strictly used during model development as a litmus test to monitor for overfitting (evident when performance on the training set significantly exceeds performance on the validation set). For this reason, the "validation data set" is also often referred to as a "development data set" in the ML literature. A validation data set does nothing to "validate" a model given information leak can occur during the training process while adjusting hyperparameters, and one can begin to overfit to the validation data set itself. Although cross-validation can help mitigate this somewhat, there is no substitute for a separate hold-out *test data set*. In order to accurately assess a given model's performance, the model *must be* evaluated on a test set that the model was not exposed to during the training process; this can either be a distinct hold-out partition from the original data set or, ideally, a completely separate, external data set. The careful choice of a testing strategy is essential for any ML approach and ideally should be developed during the planning stages of comprehensive ML projects.

CASE STUDIES IN MACHINE LEARNING
Detection of Rare Causes of Heart Failure with Preserved Ejection Fraction

The widespread adoption of EHRs and the availability of repositories of digitized cardiovascular diagnostic testing, such as echocardiograms, cardiac MRIs, and ECGs, have enabled the development of algorithms for a range of tasks, including automation of measurements (ie, left ventricular ejection fraction, diastolic dysfunction), enhancing image quality, disease diagnosis, and risk prediction for disease development or prognosis.[51–53] In HFpEF, underlying causes remain underdiagnosed, especially for rare causes, such as cardiac amyloidosis.

Several studies have examined the use different types of data to identify patients with specific causes of HFpEF. In 2018, Zhang and colleagues[54] used convolutional neural networks to train a model to accurately identify different echocardiographic views and predict specific diseases related to HFpEF (hypertrophic cardiomyopathy, cardiac amyloidosis, and pulmonary arterial hypertension) with good discrimination (C-statistics = 0.85–0.93). Tison and colleagues[55] developed a deep learning model for ECG data to predict cardiac structure and function as well as specific diseases with good discrimination for hypertrophic cardiomyopathy, cardiac amyloidosis, and pulmonary arterial hypertension (C-statistics = 0.86–0.94). Duffy and colleagues developed an end-to-end pipeline to automatically quantify left ventricular hypertrophy and predict its cause with an area under the curve of 0.83 for cardiac amyloidosis and 0.98 for hypertrophic cardiomyopathy.[56] Using ECG and echocardiographic data to identify those with cardiac amyloidosis, Goto and colleagues[57] demonstrated that the stepwise use of deep learning, initially ECG data, to identify those at high risk and then on echocardiographic data for those with increased positive predictive value from 33% to 74% to 77% in cohorts from 2 institutions. Huda and colleagues[58] trained an ML model using *International Classification of Diseases* codes to identify patients with wild-type transthyretin cardiac amyloidosis and found good to excellent performance in 4 external validation cohorts, including a large, integrated health system.

Taken together, these studies demonstrate the promise of using ML to identify rare subtypes of HFpEF on different types of data. Future areas of research for HFpEF cause detection include exploring the use of state-of-the-art NLP models, incorporating longitudinal changes in diverse data types, and fusing multiple data types into a single model. Last, although the above studies have shown promising, "in silico" results, implementation studies are needed to understand whether these technologies can be deployed to impact the care and outcomes with patients with HFpEF.

Phenomapping of Heart Failure with Preserved Ejection Fraction

Shah and colleagues[30] hypothesized that the application of ML techniques to dense phenotypic data ("phenomapping") would yield a novel classification system for HFpEF, and that the identified "pheno-groups" would have unique pathophysiologic profiles and differential outcomes. Phenotypic features used in the study included clinical variables, physical characteristics, laboratory data, ECG parameters, and echocardiographic variables. **Fig. 3** details the key steps of the study. The investigators identified 3 distinct classes (pheno-groups) of HFpEF patients with differing clinical characteristics and profiles and differential rates of cardiovascular hospitalization and death. The 3 clusters were replicated in an independent, prospective validation cohort. This approach highlights the importance of having an a priori hypothesis; using high-quality, quantitative data; and validating in a separate cohort.

Several other studies applied similar phenomapping techniques to patients with HFpEF and are reviewed in detail along with HFpEF therapeutic implications by Galli and colleagues.[59] The overlap in similar phenotypes across multiple cohorts of patients using different unsupervised learning approaches suggests that certain pheno-groups may represent a distinct pathophysiologic profile and have a differential response to therapeutics. A recent study by Pandey and colleagues[60] used deep-learning models with a limited number of echocardiographic measurements of systolic and diastolic function to characterize the severity of diastolic dysfunction and identify subgroups with differential risks of adverse events and potential response to spironolactone. For this study and other similar studies, the identification of pheno-groups should represent the starting point for future investigations, such as mechanistic studies of the underlying pathogenies of HFpEF or clinical trials testing targeted interventions. Moreover, future studies will ideally move beyond applying ML algorithms to selected groups of echocardiographic measurements to using ML to analyze the echocardiographic

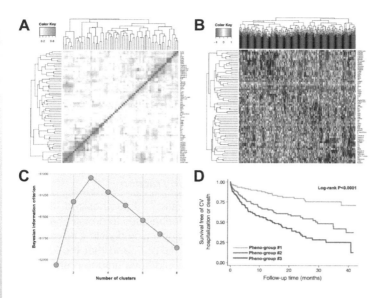

Fig. 3. Example of an unsupervised ML workflow for the identification of novel HFpEF subtypes. (*A*) The workflow for unsupervised ML begins with data processing, including examination of missing values, multiple imputation, transformation, scaling, and correlation testing, to understand the relationship between the features (variables) to be selected for the analysis. Shown here is an example of a heatmap displaying the correlation between laboratory, electrocardiographic, and echocardiographic features that were used in phenomapping of HFpEF (the color key corresponds to the range of correlation coefficients shown in the heatmap). The point of this type of analysis is to remove highly correlated features before the unsupervised learning analyses. (*B*) Next, various types of unsupervised ML analyses can be used to identify clusters within the data. In the displayed example, agglomerative hierarchical clustering was used to create an initial heatmap to demonstrate the heterogeneity of the HFpEF patients and the presence of potential clusters. (*C*) Concomitant with unsupervised learning analyses is the need to determine the optimal number of clusters. In the example shown here, model-based clustering was used on the HFpEF data set, and the optimal number of clusters was determined using the Bayesian information criterion (BIC) analyses. The lowest BIC value corresponds to 3 clusters, which is the optimal number in this example. (*D*) Once the optimal number and composition of the clusters is identified, differences in clinical characteristics, including outcomes, can be compared among the clusters. In the example shown here, the 3 HFpEF clusters differed significantly in survival free of cardiovascular hospitalization or death and represented 3 distinct clinical profiles of HFpEF. In the example shown here, pheno-group 1 was characterized by younger patients with relatively normal B-type natriuretic peptide and moderate diastolic dysfunction; pheno-group 2 included obese, diabetic patients with the worst left ventricular relaxation and high prevalence of obstructive sleep apnea; and pheno-group 3 was composed of older patients with significant right ventricular dysfunction, pulmonary hypertension, chronic kidney disease, and electrical and myocardial remodeling. CV, cardiovascular. (*Adapted from* Shah SJ, Katz DH, Selvaraj S, Burke MA, Yancy CW, Gheorghiade M, Bonow RO, Huang CC, Deo RC. Phenomapping for novel classification of heart failure with preserved ejection fraction. Circulation. 2015 Jan 20;131(3):269-79.)

images themselves, along with other types of unstructured data, such as ECGs and clinical notes, in combination with other structured demographic and clinical data. Advantages of these approaches are (1) increased throughput, reproducibility, and scalability (owing to the lack of needing human echocardiographic measurements); and (2) use of multimodal data sets, which increase likelihood of orthogonal (and therefore more informative) input features into ML models.

DISCUSSION

The authors have highlighted some of the unmet needs in HFpEF and ways in which ML may be used to address these challenges, including rare cause detection, identification of subtypes with different outcomes and potentially differential response to therapeutics, and increased efficiency for clinical trial recruitment through using NLP. Although studies using ML are becoming increasingly common in the health care field, as with any newly applied methodology, a healthy amount of skepticism is warranted. It is unlikely that ML alone will be able to solve the problem of disentangling the heterogeneity of and enhancing therapeutic targeting in HFpEF. For example, one could argue that even more important than any analytical technique is the availability of orthogonal (ie, uncorrelated) features that provide a more comprehensive viewpoint of the patients and outcomes under investigation. Furthermore, the "hype" of any new (or newly applied) analytical technique can often lead to errors in its application and interpretation, as detailed in later discussion. Finally, ML could fall prey to the lifecycle of several other novel diagnostic and analytical techniques in medicine.

Several groups have published or are in the process of developing guidelines for the design, reporting, and evaluation of ML studies in health care.[61–67] In later discussion, the authors offer

Table 1
Evaluative framework for machine learning studies

Categories	Evaluation Criteria
Study question and design	✔ Does machine learning offer specific advantages over other statistical modeling approaches? ✔ If yes, then why? Potential criteria include the data source, feature learning, outcomes, or combination of these.
Data	✔ Are data being collected primarily for (1) research or (2) clinical/administrative purposes? ✔ Are the issues of biases and data quality (ie, completeness, heterogeneity, density, accuracy, and representativeness) described and addressed?
Approach	✔ Were the reasons for the selected approaches specified (ie, supervised vs unsupervised vs semisupervised vs reinforcement learning, model selection)? ✔ If complex models are used, are we sure simpler models would not do better? Was the model chosen a priori? ✔ Is the internal validation convincing? ✔ Was the testing data set separated before model training and was there an external validation? ✔ Is the causality convincing or could features used for prediction have been produced by the outcome? ✔ Is performance properly quantified for both internal and external validation? ✔ Was the model performance compared with other models addressing the same clinical question?
Clinical relevance and generalizability	✔ Do the results have clinical relevance or provide mechanistic insight into the pathophysiology of the clinical syndrome of interest? ✔ How well should we expect the study population to generalize to the target population?

complementary recommendations to help guide future work in applying ML to HFpEF investigations (**Table 1**).

One should not apply ML algorithms to every large data set or research question; rather, one must think critically about how ML would be better than a traditional approach for the specific research question at hand. Developing a priori hypotheses and analytical plans, informed by prior research and clinical insights (from clinical domain experts), may be helpful to reduce spurious findings. For many research questions, a conventional statistical approach or study design will be sufficient. ML cannot overcome threats to validity that occur with subgroup analyses in smaller data sets or traditional, post hoc clinical trial analyses. Findings from these analyses, although potentially important, are hypothesis-generating and need to be viewed with the same level of caution as other observational studies.

Bigger data do not necessarily imply better data. First, if many of the variables included in the data set are highly correlated with each other, the addition of all these variables to the analysis is unlikely to be helpful. Orthogonal data types (ie, data that

are not highly correlated with each other and yet meaningful to the disease or outcome of interest) are essential. Second, the size of the data set cannot overcome poor data quality or bias introduced from the data or study design. For example, data from EHRs and other clinical systems are often of poor quality, incomplete, and biased.[68,69] Although longitudinal and/or multiple imputation can be used,[70,71] the missing data are likely not random. Any imputation of data or exclusion of participants with incomplete data will likely introduce bias into the results. Last, ML has the potential to detect and/or perpetuate structural racism, and there is a growing body of research on ways to ensure that ML, especially when applied in health care settings, increases equity.

Concurrent with the continued growth in the amount of data, the systems to collect, store, and organize data, and ML methods themselves, are rapidly evolving. For example, as discussed earlier, deep learning has dramatically evolved since the mid-2000s, leading to significant improvements in speech and visual object recognition.[5,29] Incorporating the latest advances in data management and ML into existing and future

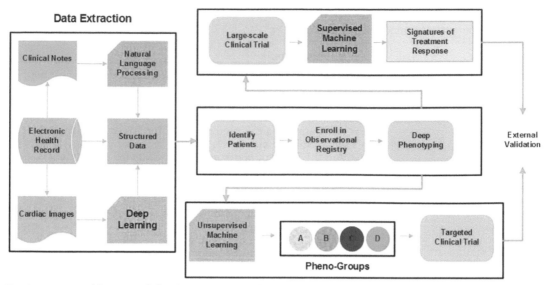

Fig. 4. Conceptual framework for the integration of ML approaches for novel classification and treatment of heterogeneous clinical syndromes, such as HF. In this precision medicine conceptual framework, 4 areas of ML discussed here (unsupervised learning, supervised learning, deep learning, and NLP) are used in combination to classify and provide targeted treatment for a heterogeneous clinical syndrome such as HF.

studies will be critical to finding meaningful application of ML to HFpEF. Large-scale HF clinical trials should be designed with ML in mind such that dense phenotypic, -omic, and physical activity (eg, accelerometer) data are collected, and training and validation subsets should be outlined in advance.

For both unsupervised and supervised ML approaches, validation in an external test data set, similar to traditional risk prediction models,[72,73] is critically important to establish the accuracy of the model. Given the fact that the ideal data sets for ML will be unique owing to the requirement for large amounts of variables from multiple domains, validation for unsupervised learning analyses will not always be immediately possible because of the lack of an appropriate test data set. However, any ML study without a test cohort should be viewed as hypothesis-generating only, with a requirement for future validation before further research of identified subgroups or integration into clinical practice.

In the case of supervised learning, validation is a requirement given the need to test the accuracy of the algorithm.[74] For supervised models, measures of discrimination and calibration should therefore be reported. Also, whenever using a complex ML algorithm, the results should be compared with those of a simpler algorithm.

In general, care must be taken in the evaluation of the quality and promise of ML algorithms. For models intended to inform clinical practice, the development of a new classification system or prediction model is not sufficient to change practice. These models must be deployed clinically, with formal testing of their performance and clinical impact; not surprisingly, the implementation of risk tools into clinical practice may not change clinical practice,[75] and additional studies for the use of ML models in clinical practice are needed, including hybrid-effectiveness studies.[76] Dataset shift" is a mismatch between the data on which the model is deployed and on which it was trained and can occur for numerous reasons, including changes in technology, the patient population, clinician behavior, or clinical workflows.[77] This mismatch can lead to change in model performance and highlights the need for a health system governance infrastructure to monitor and address model performance and impact over time.[77,78]

Future advancements in HFpEF precision medicine may require a combination of the ML techniques. Different ML approaches, such as NLP, deep learning, unsupervised ML, and supervised ML, could be used for specific tasks as part of a larger framework in order to efficiently identify novel approaches to the classification and treatment of HFpEF in clinical trials (**Fig. 4**).

SUMMARY

HFpEF is a morbid and costly clinical syndrome with significant heterogeneity. ML is an exciting tool that may help address some of the major challenges in HFpEF and in cardiovascular medicine. However, as with the application of any new technique, methodical and thoughtful application of ML to specific, hypothesis-driven questions will be essential if it is to make a lasting impact on the field of HFpEF.

DISCLOSURE

F.A. receives consulting fees from Amgen, Pfizer, and Livongo Teladoc outside of this work. S.J.S. has received research grants from the National Institutes of Health (R01 HL107577, R01 HL127028, R01 HL140731, R01 HL149423), Actelion, AstraZeneca, Corvia, Novartis, and Pfizer and has received consulting fees from Abbott, Actelion, AstraZeneca, Amgen, Aria CV, Axon Therapies, Bayer, Boehringer-Ingelheim, Boston Scientific, Bristol-Myers Squibb, Cardiora, CVRx, Cytokinetics, Edwards Lifesciences, Eidos, Eisai, Imara, Impulse Dynamics, Intellia, Ionis, Ironwood, Lilly, Merck, MyoKardia, Novartis, Novo Nordisk, Pfizer, Prothena, Regeneron, Rivus, Sanofi, Shifamed, Tenax, Tenaya, and United Therapeutics. J.T. receives consulting fees from Edwards, Abbott, GE, and Caption Health and reports spouse employment with Caption Health.

FUNDING SOURCES

Dr Ahmad was supported by grants from the Agency for Healthcare Research and Quality (K12HS026385), National Institutes of Health/National Heart, Lung, and Blood Institute (K23HL155970), and the American Heart Association (AHA number 856917). Dr Luo was supported by grants from National Institutes of Health (U01TR003528, 1R01LM013337). Dr Thomas was supported by a grant from the Irene D. Pritzker Foundation. The statements presented in this work are solely the responsibility of the author(s) and do not necessarily represent the official views of the Patient-Centered Outcomes Research Institute (PCORI), the PCORI Board of Governors or Methodology Committee, the Agency for Healthcare Research and Quality, the National Institutes of Health, or the American Heart Association.

CLINICS CARE POINTS

- Machine learning has promise to improve identifying and treating different subtypes of patients with heart failure with preserved ejection fraction but also pitfalls.

- Machine learning approaches may ultimately contribute improvements in care for patients with heart failure with preserved ejection fraction, but applications must be rigorously developed and tested before implementation into clinical care.

ACKNOWLEDGMENTS

The authors thank Mark Berendsen, MLIS and Linda O'Dwyer, MA, MSLIS, AHIP, for their assistance with the literature review for this article.

SUPPLEMENTARY DATA

Supplementary data related to this article can be found online at https://doi.org/10.1016/j.pmr.2016.04.003.

REFERENCES

1. Virani SS, Alonso A, Aparicio HJ, et al. Heart disease and stroke statistics-2021 update: a report from the American Heart Association. Circulation 2021; 143(8):e254–743.
2. Shah SJ, Kitzman DW, Borlaug BA, et al. Phenotype-specific treatment of heart failure with preserved ejection fraction: a multiorgan roadmap. Circulation 2016;134(1):73–90.
3. Murphy KP. Machine learning. Cambridge, Massachusetts: MIT Press; 2012.
4. Bishop CM. Pattern recognition and machine learning. New York: Springer; 2006.
5. Goodfellow I, Bengio Y, Courville A. Deep learning. Cambridge, MA: MIT Press; 2016.
6. Obermeyer Z, Emanuel EJ. Predicting the future - big data, machine learning, and clinical medicine. N Engl J Med 2016;375(13):1216–9.
7. Altman RB, Ashley EA. Using "big data" to dissect clinical heterogeneity. Circulation 2015;131(3): 232–3.
8. Shah SJ. Precision medicine for heart failure with preserved ejection fraction: an overview. J Cardiovasc Transl Res 2017;10(3):233–44.
9. Kittleson MM, Maurer MS, Ambardekar AV, et al. Cardiac amyloidosis: evolving diagnosis and management: a scientific statement from the American Heart Association. Circulation 2020;142(1):e7–22.
10. Kazi DS, Bellows BK, Baron SJ, et al. Cost-effectiveness of tafamidis therapy for transthyretin amyloid cardiomyopathy. Circulation 2020;141(15):1214–24.
11. Aus dem Siepen F, Hein S, Prestel S, et al. Carpal tunnel syndrome and spinal canal stenosis: harbingers of transthyretin amyloid cardiomyopathy? Clin Res Cardiol 2019;108(12):1324–30.

12. Falk RH, Alexander KM, Liao R, et al. (Light-chain) cardiac amyloidosis: a review of diagnosis and therapy. J Am Coll Cardiol 2016;68(12):1323–41.

13. Geller HI, Singh A, Alexander KM, et al. Association between ruptured distal biceps tendon and wild-type transthyretin cardiac amyloidosis. JAMA 2017; 318(10):962–3.

14. Donnelly JP, Hanna M. Cardiac amyloidosis: an update on diagnosis and treatment. Cleve Clin J Med 2017;84(12 Suppl 3):12–26.

15. Wechalekar AD, Gillmore JD, Hawkins PN. Systemic amyloidosis. Lancet 2016;387(10038): 2641–54.

16. Butler J, Fonarow GC, Zile MR, et al. Developing therapies for heart failure with preserved ejection fraction: current state and future directions. JACC Heart Fail 2014;2(2):97–112.

17. Goldstein BA, Navar AM, Carter RE. Moving beyond regression techniques in cardiovascular risk prediction: applying machine learning to address analytic challenges. Eur Heart J, 2017;38(23):1805–14.

18. Gheorghiade M, Vaduganathan M, Greene SJ, et al. Site selection in global clinical trials in patients hospitalized for heart failure: perceived problems and potential solutions. Heart Fail Rev 2014; 19(2):135–52.

19. Wehbe RM, Khan SS, Shah SJ, et al. Predicting high-risk patients and high-risk outcomes in heart failure. Heart Failure Clin 2020;16(4):387–407.

20. Adler ED, Voors AA, Klein L, et al. Improving risk prediction in heart failure using machine learning. Eur J Heart Fail 2020;22(1):139–47.

21. Greenberg B, Adler E, Campagnari C, et al. A machine learning risk score predicts mortality across the spectrum of left ventricular ejection fraction. Eur J Heart Fail 2021;23(6):995–9.

22. Zhou X, Belkin M. Chapter 22 - semi-supervised learning. In: Diniz PSR, Suykens JAK, Chellappa R, et al, editors. In signal processing, 1. Kidlington, Oxford, UK: Academic Press Library; 2014. p. 1239–69. Elsevier.

23. Sutton RS, Barto AG. Reinforcement learning: an introduction. 2nd edition. Cambridge, Massachusetts: MIT Press; 2017.

24. Vapnik V, Golowich SE, Smola A. Support vector method for function approximation, regression estimation, and signal processing. Adv Neural Inf Process Syst 1997;9:281–7.

25. Liaw A, Wiener M. Classification and regression by randomForest. R News 2002;2/3:18–22.

26. Hartigan JA, Wong MA. A k-means clustering algorithm. Appl Stat 1979;28:100–8.

27. Ng A, Jordan M, Weiss Y. On spectral clustering: analysis and an algorithm. In: Dieterich T, Becker S, Ghahramani Z, editors. Advances in neural information processing systems, 14. Cambridge: MIT Press; 2002. p. 849–56.

28. Jolliffe IT. Principal component analysis and factor analysis. In: Principal component analysis. New York, (NY): Springer New York; 1986. p. 115–28.

29. LeCun Y, Bengio Y, Hinton G. Deep learning. Nature 2015;521(7553):436–44.

30. Shah SJ, Katz DH, Selvaraj S, et al. Phenomapping for novel classification of heart failure with preserved ejection fraction. Circulation 2015;131(3):269–79.

31. Shin HC, Roth HR, Gao M, et al. Deep convolutional neural networks for computer-aided detection: CNN architectures, dataset characteristics and transfer learning. IEEE Trans Med Imaging 2016;35(5): 1285–98.

32. Hirschberg J, Manning CD. Advances in natural language processing. Science 2015;349(6245):261–6.

33. Zeng Z, Deng Y, Li X, et al. Natural language processing for EHR-based computational phenotyping. Ieee/acm Trans Comput Biol Bioinform 2019;16(1): 139–53.

34. Goldberg Y. A primer on neural network models for natural language processing. J Artif Intell Res, 57, 2016;345–420.

35. Nadkarni PM, Ohno-Machado L, Chapman WW. Natural language processing: an introduction. J Am Med Inform Assoc : JAMIA. 2011;18(5):544–51.

36. Luo Y, Thompson WK, Herr TM, et al. Natural language processing for EHR-based pharmacovigilance: a structured review. Drug Saf 2017;40(11): 1075–89.

37. Vaswani A, Shazeer NM, Parmar N, et al. Attention is all you need. ArXiv. 2017;abs/1706.03762.

38. Devlin J, Chang M-W, Lee K, Toutanova K. BERT: pre-training of deep bidirectional transformers for language understanding. Paper presented at: NAACL2019. Available at: https://aclanthology.org/N19-1423.pdf.

39. Alsentzer E, Murphy J, Boag W, et al. Publicly available clinical BERT embeddings. ArXiv. 2019;abs/1904.03323.

40. Huang K, Altosaar J, Ranganath R. ClinicalBERT: modeling clinical notes and predicting hospital readmission. ArXiv. 2019;abs/1904.05342.

41. Lee J, Yoon W, Kim S, et al. BioBERT: a pre-trained biomedical language representation model for biomedical text mining. Bioinformatics 2019;36(4): 1234–40.

42. Rasmy L, Xiang Y, Xie Z, et al. Med-BERT: pretrained contextualized embeddings on large-scale structured electronic health records for disease prediction. npj Digital Med 2021;4(1):86.

43. Brown TB, Mann B, Ryder N, et al. Language models are few-shot learners. ArXiv. 2020;abs/2005.14165.

44. Korngiebel DM, Mooney S. Considering the possibilities and pitfalls of Generative Pre-trained Transformer 3 (GPT-3) in healthcare delivery. NPJ Digital Med 2021;4.

45. Byrd RJ, Steinhubl SR, Sun J, et al. Automatic identification of heart failure diagnostic criteria, using text analysis of clinical notes from electronic health records. Int J Med Inf 2014;83(12):983–92.

46. Friedlin J, McDonald CJ. A natural language processing system to extract and code concepts relating to congestive heart failure from chest radiology reports. AMIA Annu Symp Proc 2006; 269–73. Annual Symposium Proceedings/AMIA Symposium.

47. Ho JC, Ghosh J, Steinhubl SR, et al. Limestone: high-throughput candidate phenotype generation via tensor factorization. J Biomed Inform 2014;52: 199–211.

48. Peissig PL, Santos Costa V, Caldwell MD, et al. Relational machine learning for electronic health record-driven phenotyping. J Biomed Inform 2014;52: 260–70.

49. Vijayakrishnan R, Steinhubl SR, Ng K, et al. Prevalence of heart failure signs and symptoms in a large primary care population identified through the use of text and data mining of the electronic health record. J Card Fail 2014;20(7):459–64.

50. Schölkopf B, Smola AJ. Learning with Kernels: support vector machines, regularization, optimization, and beyond. Cambridge: MIT Press; 2001.

51. Litjens G, Ciompi F, Wolterink JM, et al. State-of-the-art deep learning in cardiovascular image analysis. JACC: Cardiovasc Imaging 2019;12(8_Part_1): 1549–65.

52. Seetharam K, Brito D, Farjo PD, et al. The role of artificial intelligence in cardiovascular imaging: state of the art review. Front Cardiovasc Med 2020;7(374).

53. Luo Y, Mao C, Yang Y, et al. Integrating hypertension phenotype and genotype with hybrid non-negative matrix factorization. Bioinformatics 2019;35(16): 2885.

54. Zhang J, Gajjala S, Agrawal P, et al. Fully automated echocardiogram interpretation in clinical practice. Circulation 2018;138(16):1623–35.

55. Tison GH, Zhang J, Delling FN, et al. Automated and interpretable patient ECG profiles for disease detection, tracking, and discovery. Circ Cardiovasc Qual Outcomes 2019;12(9):e005289.

56. Duffy G, Cheng P, Yuan N, et al. High-throughput precision phenotyping of left ventricular hypertrophy with cardiovascular deep learning. ArXiv. 2021;abs/2106.12511.

57. Goto S, Mahara K, Beussink-Nelson L, et al. Artificial intelligence-enabled fully automated detection of cardiac amyloidosis using electrocardiograms and echocardiograms. Nat Commun 2021;12(1):2726.

58. Huda A, Castaño A, Niyogi A, et al. A machine learning model for identifying patients at risk for wild-type transthyretin amyloid cardiomyopathy. Nat Commun 2021;12(1):2725.

59. Galli E, Bourg C, Kosmala W, et al. Phenomapping heart failure with preserved ejection fraction using machine learning cluster analysis: prognostic and therapeutic implications. Heart Failure Clin 2021; 17(3):499–518.

60. Pandey A, Kagiyama N, Yanamala N, et al. Deep-learning models for the echocardiographic assessment of diastolic dysfunction. JACC Cardiovasc Imaging 2021;14(10):1887–900.

61. Collins GS, Dhiman P, Andaur Navarro CL, et al. Protocol for development of a reporting guideline (TRIPOD-AI) and risk of bias tool (PROBAST-AI) for diagnostic and prognostic prediction model studies based on artificial intelligence. BMJ Open 2021; 11(7):e048008.

62. Liu Y, Chen P-HC, Krause J, et al. How to read articles that use machine learning: users' guides to the medical literature. JAMA 2019;322(18): 1806–16.

63. Sengupta PP, Shrestha S, Berthon B, et al. Proposed requirements for cardiovascular imaging-related machine learning evaluation (PRIME): a checklist: reviewed by the American College of Cardiology Healthcare Innovation Council. JACC: Cardiovasc Imaging 2020;13(9):2017–35.

64. Vasey B, Clifton DA, Collins GS, et al. DECIDE-AI: new reporting guidelines to bridge the development-to-implementation gap in clinical artificial intelligence. Nat Med 2021;27(2):186–7.

65. Stevens LM, Mortazavi BJ, Deo RC, et al. Recommendations for reporting machine learning analyses in clinical research. Circ Cardiovasc Qual Outcomes 2020;13(10):e006556.

66. Liu X, Faes L, Calvert MJ, et al. Extension of the CONSORT and SPIRIT statements. Lancet 2019; 394(10205):1225.

67. Norgeot B, Quer G, Beaulieu-Jones BK, et al. Minimum information about clinical artificial intelligence modeling: the MI-CLAIM checklist. Nat Med 2020; 26(9):1320–4.

68. Bae CJ, Griffith S, Fan Y, et al. The challenges of data quality evaluation in a joint data warehouse. EGEMS (Wash DC) 2015;3(1):1125.

69. Hersh WR, Weiner MG, Embi PJ, et al. Caveats for the use of operational electronic health record data in comparative effectiveness research. Med Care 2013;51(8 Suppl 3):S30–7.

70. Wells BJ, Chagin KM, Nowacki AS, et al. Strategies for handling missing data in electronic health record derived data. EGEMS (Wash DC) 2013;1(3):1035.

71. Luo Y, Szolovits P, Dighe AS, et al. 3D-MICE: integration of cross-sectional and longitudinal imputation for multi-analyte longitudinal clinical data. J Am Med Inform Assoc 2018;25(6):645–53.

72. Lloyd-Jones DM. Cardiovascular risk prediction: basic concepts, current status, and future directions. Circulation 2010;121(15):1768–77.

73. Steyerberg EW, Moons KG, van der Windt DA, et al. Prognosis Research Strategy (PROGRESS) 3: prognostic model research. Plos Med 2013;10(2): e1001381.

74. Saeb S, Lonini L, Jayaraman A, et al. The need to approximate the use-case in clinical machine learning. GigaScience, May 2017;6(5):1–9.

75. Peiris D, Usherwood T, Panaretto K, et al. Effect of a computer-guided, quality improvement program for cardiovascular disease risk management in primary health care: the treatment of cardiovascular risk using electronic decision support cluster-randomized trial. Circ Cardiovasc Qual Outcomes 2015;8(1): 87–95.

76. Curran GM, Bauer M, Mittman B, et al. Effectiveness-implementation hybrid designs: combining elements of clinical effectiveness and implementation research to enhance public health impact. Med Care 2012; 50(3):217–26.

77. Finlayson SG, Subbaswamy A, Singh K, et al. The clinician and dataset shift in artificial intelligence. N Engl J Med 2021;385(3):283–6.

78. Guo LL, Pfohl SR, Fries J, et al. Systematic review of approaches to preserve machine learning performance in the presence of temporal dataset shift in clinical medicine. Appl Clin Inform 2021;12(4): 808–15.

Artificial Intelligence and Mechanical Circulatory Support

Song Li, MD[a], Gavin W. Hickey, MD[b], Matthew M. Lander, MD[c],
Manreet K. Kanwar, MD[c],*

KEYWORDS

- Artificial intelligence • Machine learning • Mechanical circulatory support • Heart failure

KEY POINTS

- Artificial intelligence/machine learning has shown promising results in identifying patients appropriate for mechanical circulatory support therapy, predicting risks after mechanical circulatory support device implantation, and monitoring for adverse events.
- State-of-the-art machine learning algorithms, leveraging new data sources, stand to further expand artificial intelligence capabilities in mechanical circulatory support.
- Clinical implementation of artificial intelligence in mechanical circulatory support has been very limited.
- An interdisciplinary workforce is needed to demonstrate artificial intelligence's clinical efficacy, reliability, transparency, and equity to drive implementation.

HISTORY

Alan Turing initially explored the mathematical possibility of artificial intelligence (AI) in his 1950 paper, Computing Machinery and Intelligence, in which he conceptually discussed how to build intelligent machines[1]. In 1956, the logic theorist was designed as a program to mimic the problem-solving skills of a human and presented at the Dartmouth Summer Research Project on AI. This work catalyzed the next 2 decades of AI research, which was marked by multiple success stories and setbacks. One of the biggest setbacks was the lack of computational power for the substantial needs of AI, at the time. In the 1980s, AI was reignited by an expansion of algorithmic tools—deep learning techniques, which allowed computers to learn using experience and mimic the decision-making process of a human expert.

However, it was only in the 1990s and 2000s that several landmark goals of AI were achieved. These included spoken language interpretation and an increase in computer storage limits, as well as processing speeds. This has heralded the age of "big data"—an age where we have the capacity to collect huge sums of information and apply AI to advance the fields of technology, banking, marketing, and entertainment, as well as medicine.

In recent years, there has been a significant increase in medical research using applications of various aspects of AI, especially in cardiovascular medicine. Physicians have long needed to identify, quantify, correlate, and process complex relationships among various data and patient outcomes. There is increasing demand to provide faster, more personalized care, lower costs, and decrease hospital readmissions and mortality by using sophisticated algorithms that can process

[a] Division of Cardiology, University of Washington, 1959 Northeast Pacific Street, Seattle, WA 98195, USA; [b] Division of Cardiology, University of Pittsburgh School of Medicine, 200 Lothrop Street, PUH, 5B, Pittsburgh, PA 15213, USA; [c] Cardiovascular Institute, Allegheny Health Network, 320 E North Avenue, Pittsburgh, PA 15212, USA
* Corresponding author.
E-mail address: Manreet.KANWAR@ahn.org
Twitter: @lisong2003 (S.L.); @GavHick (G.W.H.); @MattLanderMD (M.M.L.); @manreetkanwar (M.K.K.)

Heart Failure Clin 18 (2022) 301–309
https://doi.org/10.1016/j.hfc.2021.11.005
1551-7136/22/© 2021 Elsevier Inc. All rights reserved.

patterns from large datasets. AI has the potential to exploit increasingly available large datasets in advancing patient care. It is hoped that AI will simplify the practices and processes of health care by performing tasks that are typically done by humans, but in less time and more economically. Initially dismissed by many as purely theoretical, with little potential on clinical workflow or patient care, AI in health care is projected to reach a $150 billion valuation in the next 5 years.[2]

RELEVANCE

People who suffer from end-stage heart failure (HF) face debilitating symptoms, frequent hospitalizations, and high medical costs.[3–5] Mechanical circulatory support (MCS) such as durable left ventricular assist device (LVAD) is a therapy proven to improve quality of life and mortality in patients with end-stage HF.[6–8] From early recognition of disease progression, to establishment of LVAD candidacy to the postoperative period, there are numerous areas where complex decision-making is necessary. AI is uniquely suited for application in this field.

Estimates are that those implanted with durable LVADs are only a fraction of those potentially eligible. There is an under-recognition of these patients as they suffer through the vicious cycle of end-stage HF. This situation may be expected when advanced HF expertise is concentrated at large referral centers while many potential LVAD candidates present and re-present at smaller community hospitals. Although there is a dearth of advanced HF–trained cardiologists to a have meaningful impact on timely recognition and referral of patients with end-stage HF, AI can help. Systems can be created whereby AI allows automatic detection of cardiogenic shock or "frequent flyer" readmissions and recommends referral to a tertiary care center. Similarly, community hospitals may not have the training to provide appropriate care to a patient on MCS who arrives emergently, something with which AI can also assist.

Although recent LVAD technology advances have improved outcomes, adverse event rates remain unacceptably high.[9] This factor places an emphasis on the appropriate timing of therapy to maximize benefit and minimize harm to the patient. Assessment of the LVAD candidate is important both to support the patient's acceptance and understanding but also to prognosticate their perioperative risk. Another important element of candidacy is the preoperative assessment of the patient's right ventricle (RV). Current risk scores and diagnostic tools have proven limited in accurately predicting postoperative right ventricular failure.[10–13] There are often innumerable data points to select from, including echocardiography, cardiac catheterization, and laboratory studies. The relationships and associations these data may or may not have with outcomes lends itself to the use of AI as a powerful tool to provide clarity in RV failure prediction.

An electronic device such as an LVAD that generates extensive data every minute is a distinctive opportunity for AI to understand, predict, and hopefully decrease adverse events. This constant stream of information is ripe to be transformed into actionable algorithms for both the patient and LVAD team. Full automation—an integrated LVAD AI system—has the potential to revolutionize quality of life and clinical outcomes, as it manages alarming trends on the go and intercedes before harm is incurred.

MACHINE LEARNING TECHNIQUES

AI is a term that broadly describes methods that allow computers to complete functions typically done by humans.[14] Machine learning (ML) describes numerous computerized techniques that generate a predictive model from an algorithm and data. The typical workflow for an ML algorithm is data input followed by model training and testing, and finally the output comprising the predictions made.[15] An ML model needs to be "properly learned" to be effective, meaning that predictions are accurate with both training and testing data. If a trained ML model loses accuracy on new data, it is said to be overfit.[16] Conversely, a model that does not accurately predict training data is underfit, usually occurring when a model is too simplistic. Data quality can also affect model performance; excessive, heterogeneous, or missing data points can all negatively impact output accuracy.

Supervised and unsupervised learning are the 2 main categories of ML.[15] Supervised learning is done when the sample is labeled, for example, when the desired output is known in the training data. Unsupervised methods are applied if the data are unlabeled. Patterns are, therefore, derived from the input data to create groups, such as in hierarchical clustering or principal components analysis. By identifying similar groups in the input data, new relationships and connections can be made. The output of unsupervised ML can even be entered into a supervised approach, which takes the new input and can train a model to make accurate predictions. A semisupervised approach can infer labels from a small amount of labeled data for a large amount of unlabeled data, allowing for better performance and lower costs. Ensemble learning allows for the combination of multiple models that may identify different patterns into one more robust prediction algorithm.

As computing technology improves, so do the capabilities of ML. Deep learning describes methods that use neural network layers to achieve the desired output. The most basic neural network has 3 layers: an input layer, a hidden layer, and an output layer. However, a deep neural network can have multiple hidden layers that can sequentially analyze and transform the input data into unique patterns not achievable by other techniques. More complicated networks allow for the algorithm to learn and minimize error via a process called back propagation.[17] Training such a system generally requires very large datasets, owing to the numerous hidden layers. There is also a black box–like effect with these methods as interpreting the prediction is challenged by the complex and hidden process that creates the output.

Today, there are many innovative applications of ML to the field of medicine. Computer vision has recently evolved exponentially as computing power has improved and ML has matured. It encompasses the use of ML (often neural networks) to allow for the perception of visual stimuli, which may translate into detection, classification, or localization.[18] The obvious applications are to radiology, pathology, and so on, to detect patterns that may otherwise be missed by even the most experienced clinicians, improving diagnostic performance.[19–21] Strokes can be found, cancers screened for, and even COVID-19 detection models have been developed.[22–24] In cardiology specifically, computer vision can be trained to classify pulmonary hypertension, cardiac amyloid, and hypertrophic cardiomyopathy from echocardiographic images.[25,26]

As discussed elsewhere in this article, ML algorithms require very large datasets when multilayered and complex networks are created. Changing the distribution of a model often necessitates the creation of another large training dataset, which can be logistically challenging and expensive. Transfer learning allows for the retention of the knowledge extracted from a previously trained algorithm to be conveyed to a new model without having to go through retraining from scratch. For example, a neural network already trained for classification of chest radiographs may be able to be successfully applied to COVID-19 pneumonia recognition via transfer learning.[27] These techniques can leverage complex ML networks trained on large datasets and apply them to similar but different domains and yet maintain performance.

Bidirectional encoder representations from transformers is a newer model developed by researchers at Google AI Language.[28] It is a major step forward in ML as it applies to natural language processing (NLP). By reading a sequence of words in a nondirectional manner with attention mechanism, the model can learn the context of a word from what surrounds it. Through a process called fine tuning, the model can be trained to achieve predictive performance never previously attained. The applications are myriad; bidirectional encoder representations from transformers techniques can be used to deploy powerful data extraction to electronic health records (EHR), enabling highly accurate chart review efforts.[29]

CLINICAL APPLICATIONS

In recent years, with the exponential growth of AI research in medicine, there has been a wide range of AI/ML applications in various MCS-related fields (**Fig. 1**). In this review, we attempt to delineate the applications of AI/ML in MCS from 2 different angles. One angle categorizes the various AI/ML applications by their intended clinical purposes. In the literature thus far, AI/ML has been used to risk stratify patients with HF to identify high-risk patients appropriate for MCS therapy, predict outcomes after MCS device implantation, and monitor MCS patients for adverse events. The other angle analyzes current AI/ML applications from a technical aspect, focusing on innovations in ML algorithms and model performance compared with traditional statistics. From this angle, AI/ML applications in MCS have used a variety of cutting-edge tree-based, Bayesian, and neural network models. It is also important to note 2 ML specializations that are unique to medicine and to MCS: medical audio/image analysis and EHR analysis.

Clinical Perspective

Beginning with the clinical perspective, the first area AI/ML can aid MCS therapy is to better identify high-risk patients with HF to be evaluated for MCS therapy. The optimal timing of advanced HF therapy referral for ambulatory outpatients is still unclear and, despite available clinical support tools, many patients are still referred too late. Many patients, especially in rural areas, may also lack access to health care providers familial with MCS therapy. Although patients with acute cardiogenic shock are more readily identifiable, the decision to and the timing of transfer to a hospital with a higher level of available MCS therapy are also not well-known.

In this area, some recent research studies are laying the foundation for AI/ML to play an active role in the future. In 2017, Choi and colleagues[30] applied a neural network to a large EHR database to predict the incidence of HF 12 to 18 months in

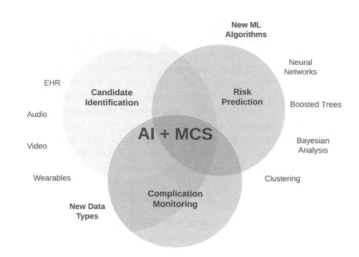

Fig. 1. Areas of applications of AI/ML in MCS. EHR, electronic health record.

the future and achieved an area under the curve (AUC) of 0.883, which represented a significant improvement from logistic regression. Later studies applied ML algorithm to predict mortality risk in large HF cohorts. Adler and colleagues[31] applied a boosted decision tree algorithm (Ada-Boost) to a cohort of patients with HF identified by querying the EHR and achieved higher accuracy (AUC, 0.88) than 3 traditional risk models (AUC, 0.63–0.78) in predicting mortality risk. Greenberg and colleagues[32] tested the same ML model across the spectrum of left ventricular ejection fraction and found similarly good risk discrimination in patients with HF with a reduced, midrange, or preserved left ventricular ejection fraction (AUC, 0.83–0.89). Similarly, Jing and colleagues[33] applied a boosted tree-based model (XGBoost) to a large EHR database with 26,971 patients with HF and 276,819 clinical episodes and achieved an AUC of 0.77 for 1-year all-cause mortality. However, in this study the best ML model only slightly outperformed linear logistic regression (AUC, 0.74). In addition to stratifying mortality risk in patients with HF to identify high-risk patients for MCS therapy and/or heart transplantation, it is also possible to train an ML model to predict the need for AHFT directly. Among patients with advanced HF in the Registry Evaluation of Vital Information for VADs in Ambulatory Life (REVIVAL) registry, Yao and colleagues[34] combined fuzzy set theory and neural network to predict the need for MCS or urgent heart transplant listing, and achieved excellent, yet only slightly better, model discrimination than logistic regression (AUC, 0.838 vs AUC, 0.812). ML has also been shown to achieve excellent mortality risk discrimination in the setting of acute HF.[35]

The second area where AI/ML has been frequently applied is predicting risk after implantation of MCS devices. Knowing the likelihood of adverse events after MCS implantation allows clinicians to select patients most likely to benefit from MCS therapy and to potentially adopt strategies to decrease the risk of predicted adverse events. The research group of Antaki and colleagues has been playing a leading role in this area, using data from the Interagency Registry for Mechanically Assisted Circulatory Support (INTERMACS) to predict adverse events after durable LVAD implantation.[36–39] Their Bayesian models were able to predict 12-month mortality with an AUC of 0.70 and right ventricular failure with AUCs between 0.83 and 0.90 for different time points.[36,37] A unique advantage of Bayesian models compared with other ML models is that Bayesian models are inherently explainable, both on a global (model) level and on a local (individual prediction) level. The ability to explain the inner workings of an ML model, compared with operating within a black box, is key to implementation of AI/ML in medicine, and will be discussed in more detail later. Other decision tree–based ML algorithms have also been tested to predict mortality after LVAD implantation with similarly good results.[40,41] ML approaches allow for an improved visualization and understanding of adverse events burden after LVAD implantation.[42] Two unique innovations in this area include an ML clustering analysis to identify sequential patterns of adverse events in patients with an LVAD[39] and a neural network model directly trained on echocardiogram videos to predict RV failure after LVAD implantation, which outperformed 2 traditional clinical risk models (AUC, 0.729 vs ACU, 0.605–0.616).[43]

A third area in MCS where AI/ML has been applied is the monitoring of adverse events in patients after MCS device implantation. In this area, the first published application dates back to 1995 when Stöcklmayer and colleagues[44] applied a neural network model to a rotary blood pump in vitro to estimate left atrial pressure and identify suction and near-suction states. More recently, researchers have demonstrated the ability to use LVAD waveforms to predict impending pump failure in the HeartMate XVE LVAD and to identify cardiac arrhythmias in the Debakey LVAD.[45,46] Real-life out-of-hospital telemonitoring of patients with an LVAD has also been attempted in a cohort of 11 patients implanted with the HeartAssist 5 and acute VAD LVADs, which offer telemetric monitoring capabilities.[47] A total of 6216 alarm messages, mostly low-flow alarms owing to hypovolemia and suspected pump thrombosis, were received over a total of 2438 patient-days of follow-up. Manually reviewing all the alarms would certainly overwhelm the human resources of a typical VAD clinic; thus, AI is urgently needed to better identify high-risk alarm conditions needing urgent human attention. Telemonitoring using a wearable sensor has also been tested in ambulatory patients with HF to predict HF hospitalization. The LINK-HF study used a custom multisensor patch that collects continuous electrocardiograph waveform, 3-axis accelerometry, skin impedance, skin temperature, and information on activity and posture, and applied an ML similarity-based modeling to establish individualized physiologic baselines and detect deviations from the baseline.[48] The physiologic deviations were able to predict HF hospitalizations with 76% to 88% sensitivity and 85% specificity at a median of 6.5 days before hospitalization. It would be very interesting to see if a similar multisensor patch or, better yet, built-in sensors in future LVADs, can enable early detection of clinical decompensation.

Technical Perspective

From an ML technical perspective, AI/ML applications in MCS can be categorized into 2 main areas. One branch of research has strived to achieve better risk prediction by applying new ML algorithms and models to traditional datasets. The underlying logic is that traditional statistical models, such as frequently used linear and logistic regression models, are inadequate because they, in their basic forms, do not capture nonlinear relationships and variable interactions well. It is posited that MCS-related problems often have these complex relationships that are better modeled by more flexible ML algorithms such as decision-tree–based models (random forest, boosted trees), Bayesian

models, and neural networks. Many of the examples discussed elsewhere in this article fall into this category.[31–33,36–38,40,41,49] Unsupervised ML is another example of applying new algorithms to existing datasets to gain new insights. In this regard, unsupervised clustering algorithms have been applied to traditional registry datasets to identify sequential patterns of adverse events in patients with an LVAD and to identify phenotypes of patients with cardiogenic shock, many of whom received temporary MCS devices.[39,50]

Another branch of research applies ML algorithms to new data sources that are difficult to incorporate into traditional statistical models. EHR and audiovisual data are 2 prime examples. Non-ML research has leveraged EHRs by automatically querying tabular data from the EHR instead of manual data collection. However, truly incorporating the multimodal and longitudinal features of the EHR has only been feasible with recent advances in NLP and artificial neural networks. For example, Choi and colleagues[30] used recurrent neural networks on longitudinal EHR data to predict incident HF. Zhang and colleagues[51] used NLP methods to identify New York Heart Association functional class from unstructured clinical notes in the EHR. Recent advances in transformer deep learning model using attention mechanism have been adopted for the EHR and is a promising tool for MCS applications.[52]

Applications of AI/ML, especially deep neural networks, for audiovisual data also have great potential for MCS, because as the field is heavily dependent on acoustic and videographic information for decision-making. Electrocardiographs, echocardiograms, LVAD waveforms, LVAD sounds, and LVAD driveline exit site appearance are all potential data sources for AI/ML applications. Echocardiogram videos have been used directly to assess RV function, predict RV failure after LVAD implantation, and LVAD sound has been used to identify significant aortic regurgitation with good accuracy (AUC, 0.73).[43,53–56] A group of innovative researchers applied convolutional neural network models to LVAD driveline photographs to identify driveline wound infections with an accuracy similar to human experts.[57] These types of AI/ML applications would allow patients to monitor the status of their LVADs closely from the convenience of their homes and have the potential to significantly decrease mortality and morbidity in patients with MCS devices.

LIMITATIONS AND ONGOING ADVANCEMENT

A combination of availability of large datasets and rapid technological advances in computing power has led to the increased uptake and use of ML in multiple aspects of health care. However, there are some important limitations of AI for medical applications in general and in the field of MCS.

ML is data hungry, generally requiring much larger datasets than traditional statistics. An incredible amount of health data is now being generated, estimated at 10^{18} bytes from 2019 in the United States alone and growing at 48% annually.[58] Yet, the creation of large medical datasets still often relies on manual extraction of variables from the EHR and data labeling by human experts. Time-consuming and inherently biased by variable selection, this process is being vastly improved by recent advances. New interoperable EHR data structure such as fast health care interoperability resources and improvement in NLP now allow tens of thousands of data points be extracted for each patient with little human intervention. Using these methods on an EHR database of 216,221 patients, a research team from Google was able to extract more than 48 billion data points for ML modeling.[59] Having access to all available data points may allow ML algorithms to discover previously unknown but clinically relevant variables. However, this process can be computationally expensive, and the resultant models may be too slow for point-of-care use.

In addition to traditional EHRs, cloud-based platforms have been created. One such example of a large cloud based data marketplace is the American Heart Association Precision Medicine Platform.[60] In partnership with Amazon Web Services, the goal in its creation is to enhance and investigate the area of precision medicine via ML and big data. This and other large registries will be instrumental in allowing broader application of ML in health care.

Another significant limitation for AI use in MCS is the limited number of patients implanted. Data from the STS-INTERMACS annual report include 25,551 patients implanted with a continuous flow LVAD from 2010 to 2019.[61] Although the STS-INTERMACS registry has a relatively large number of patients, the registry lacks granularity and is relatively heterogeneous, with data from 3 different types of continuous flow LVADs and at least 2 different surgical approaches (sternotomy and thoracotomy). Of the 25,551 LVADs implanted, only 15% (3901) were of the most contemporary LVAD still being implanted. Newer ML techniques such as transfer learning may prove immensely helpful to improve model performance when the sample size is small.

Despite advances in AI/ML, there are many examples of ML algorithms not performing better than traditional models. In an analysis on prediction of HF outcomes there was minimal improvement in ML over traditional logistic regression models.[62] A recent systematic review of ML compared with logistic regression for binary outcomes showed no benefit for ML over logistic regression.[63] Whether the sometimes mediocre performance of ML is due to the inherent noise and bias in the underlying datasets or can be improved with better ML algorithms remains to be seen.

Another limitation to the clinical use and acceptance of ML is the lack of transparency, the black box component of ML. Some of this reluctance can be attributed to a lack of understanding of ML and AI in general among the health care community, which can lead to mistrust of ML models and therefore a lack of use. In 1 instance, an early warning system for septic shock was developed using an ML algorithm. Despite excellent predictive accuracy, nurses and physicians did not find it useful clinically. Specifically, clinicians tended to trust their intuition over seemingly complex predictive algorithms.[64] One solution for the lack of transparency and interpretability is the use of explainable ML methods. For example, Shapley additive explanations (SHAP) is a unified framework that allows for more interpretable ML models.[65] SHAP values provide the estimated impact of each variable in the model as well as whether the effect is positive or negative. The use of SHAP provided valuable insights into the importance of each variable in a recent paper using ML to predict acute kidney injury after cardiac surgery.[66] The further development and use of explainable ML methods such as SHAP will likely improve the acceptance of ML models in clinical settings by both clinicians and patients.

INCORPORATION INTO CLINICAL PRACTICE

In the last 2 decades, there has been an explosion of AI applications in nearly all industries and all facets of life. The adoption of AI in medicine has tremendous promise in fulfilling the quadruple aims of modern health care systems, namely, improving the experience of care, improving the health of populations, decreasing per capita costs, and improving the work–life of health care providers.[67] However, even though AI/ML research in medicine has accelerated to more than 16,000 publications in 2020 in the MEDLINE database, the implementation of AI in routine clinical use has been scantly reported.[68] Health care professionals are key stakeholders to evaluate barriers and define strategies to drive AI implementation in medicine. To achieve this goal, an interdisciplinary workforce is needed to integrate the expertise of health care providers, AI/ML developers, health system leaders, ethicists, and patients. A cross-disciplinary curriculum must be developed and deployed so that health care providers can assess and correctly use AI products and services akin to other medical products. Vice versa, such curriculum can empower AI/ML developers to build AI products that adhere to the safety, efficacy, and ethical principles of health care. Having a shared knowledge base and language is critical to effective collaboration in such interdisciplinary health AI teams.

In addition to an interdisciplinary health AI workforce, another key barrier to implementing health AI products is ensuring the quality of the AI products. Health AI products are different from traditional medical treatments or devices where safety and efficacy are the 2 primary considerations. Although the standards of testing for health AI products are still being hotly debated among developers, users, investors, and regulators, it is clear that health AI products require testing in new domains. However, first and foremost, similar to other medical products, health AI products need to show improvement not only in statistical accuracy, but also in clinical outcomes. A second and related domain is reliability, which means that AI models need to be generalizable to a reasonable extent, for example, to function well in different patient populations, locations, and over time. There should be built-in or external quality assessment tools that can monitor model performance with new data inputs or better yet incorporate new data to improve performance. A third domain is transparency and explainability. Transparency means that sufficient information about the design of AI products should be available to allow end users and the public to assess the quality of the AI models. Explainability allows clinicians and patients to understand the factors behind AI models' results and is key to inspire confidence and trust. The last domain is ethics. AI models should be derived from diverse datasets representative of the disease population and scrutinized of underlying biases in data. Explainability can be very helpful to show that the inner workings of AI models do not bias against certain groups of patients. When built and used correctly, AI models could significantly decrease existing bias and inequalities in health care.

CLINICS CARE POINTS

- When evaluating AI/ML algorithms for clinical applications, pay close attention to whether the algorithms have been externally validated, tested in applicable and inclusive patient populations, and have reasonable transparency.

- Partner with ML/AI data scientists and consider participation in clinical trials that evaluate AI/ML products.

DISCLOSURE

M.K. Kanwar serves on the Advisory Board for Abiomed. S. Li, G.W. Hickey, and M.M. Lander have nothing to disclose.

REFERENCES

1. Turing AM. I.—Computing machinery and intelligence. Mind 1950;LIX(236):433–60.
2. Bohr A, Memarzadeh K. The rise of artificial intelligence in healthcare applications. In: Bohr A, Memarzadeh K, editors. Artificial intelligence in healthcare. Cambridge, MA: Academic Press; 2020. p. 25–60.
3. Ambrosy AP, Fonarow GC, Butler J, et al. The global health and economic burden of hospitalizations for heart failure: lessons learned from hospitalized heart failure registries. J Am Coll Cardiol 2014;63:1123–33.
4. Benjamin EJ, Virani SS, Callaway CW, et al. Heart disease and stroke statistics-2018 update: a report from the American Heart Association. Circulation 2018;137:e67–492.
5. Ni H, Xu J. Recent trends in heart failure-related mortality: United States, 2000-2014. NCHS Data Brief 2015;(231):1–8.
6. Rogers JG, Pagani FD, Tatooles AJ, et al. Intrapericardial left ventricular assist device for advanced heart failure. N Engl J Med 2017;376(5):451–60.
7. Slaughter MS, Rogers JG, Milano CA, et al. Advanced heart failure treated with continuous-flow left ventricular assist device. N Engl J Med 2009; 361:2241–51.
8. Rose EA, Gelijns AC, Moskowitz AJ, et al. Long-term use of a left ventricular assist device for end-stage heart failure. N Engl J Med 2001;345:1435–43.
9. Mehra MR, Uriel N, Naka Y, et al. A fully magnetically levitated left ventricular assist device - final report. N Engl J Med 2019;380(17):1618–27.
10. Morine KJ, Kiernan MS, Pham DT, et al. Pulmonary artery pulsatility index is associated with right ventricular failure after left ventricular assist device surgery. J Card Fail 2016;22:110–6.
11. Matthews JC, Koelling TM, Pagani FD, et al. The right ventricular failure risk score: a pre-operative tool for assessing the risk of right ventricular failure in left ventricular assist device candidates. J Am Coll Cardiol 2008;51:2163–72.
12. Kormos RL, Teuteberg JJ, Pagani FD, et al. Right ventricular failure in patients with the HeartMate II continuous-flow left ventricular assist device: incidence,

risk factors, and effect on outcomes. J Thorac Cardiovasc Surg 2010;139(5):1316–24.

13. Drakos SG, Janicki L, Horne BD, et al. Risk factors predictive of right ventricular failure after left ventricular assist device implantation. Am J Cardiol 2010; 105:1030–5.

14. Johnson KW, Soto JT, Glicksberg BS, et al. Artificial intelligence in cardiology. J Am Coll Cardiol 2018; 71(23):2668–79.

15. Camacho DM, Collins KM, Powers RK, et al. Next-generation machine learning for biological networks. Cell 2018;173:1581–92.

16. Domingos P. A few useful things to know about machine learning. Commun ACM 2012;55:78–87.

17. LeCun Y, Bengio Y, Hinton G. Deep learning. Nature 2015;521(7553):436–44.

18. Esteva A, Chou K, Yeung S, et al. Deep learning-enabled medical computer vision. NPJ Digit Med 2021;4:5.

19. Singh SP, Wang L, Gupta S, et al. 3D deep learning on medical images: a review. Sensors 2020;20: 5097.

20. Christiansen EM, Yang SJ, Ando DM, et al. In silico labeling: predicting fluorescent labels in unlabeled images. Cell 2018;173:792–803.e9.

21. Ting DSW, Pasquale LR, Peng L, et al. Artificial intelligence and deep learning in ophthalmology. Br J Ophthalmol 2019;103:167–75.

22. Chilamkurthy S, Ghosh R, Tanamala S, et al. Deep learning algorithms for detection of critical findings in head CT scans: a retrospective study. Lancet 2018;392:2388–96.

23. Chen PHC, Gadepalli K, MacDonald R, et al. An augmented reality microscope with real-time artificial intelligence integration for cancer diagnosis. Nat Med 2019;25:1453–7.

24. Zhang J, Xie Y, Pang G, et al. Viral pneumonia screening on chest X-Rays using confidence-aware anomaly detection. IEEE Trans Med Imaging 2020;40(3):879–90.

25. Zhang J, Gajjala S, Agrawal P, et al. Fully automated echocardiogram interpretation in clinical practice: feasibility and diagnostic accuracy. Circulation 2018;138:1623–35.

26. Ghorbani A, Ouyang D, Abid A, et al. Deep learning interpretation of echocardiograms. NPJ Digit Med 2020;3:1–10.

27. Apostolopoulos ID, Mpesiana TA. Covid-19: automatic detection from x-ray images utilizing transfer learning with convolutional neural networks. Phys Eng Sci Med 2020;43:635–40.

28. Devlin J, Chang MW, Lee K, et al. Bert: pre-training of deep bidirectional transformers for language understanding. arXiv; 2018.

29. Li F, Jin Y, Liu W, et al. Fine-tuning bidirectional encoder representations from transformers (BERT)–based models on large-scale electronic health record notes: an empirical study. JMIR Med Inform 2019;7:e14830.

30. Choi E, Schuetz A, Stewart WF, et al. Using recurrent neural network models for early detection of heart failure onset. J Am Med Inform Assoc 2017;24(2): 361–70.

31. Adler ED, Voors AA, Klein L, et al. Improving risk prediction in heart failure using machine learning. Eur J Heart Fail 2020;22(1):139–47.

32. Greenberg B, Adler E, Campagnari C, et al. A machine learning risk score predicts mortality across the spectrum of left ventricular ejection fraction. Eur J Heart Fail 2021;23(6):995–9.

33. Jing L, Cerna AEU, Good CW, et al. A machine learning approach to management of heart failure populations. JACC Heart Fail 2020;8(7): 578–87.

34. Yao H, Aaronson KD, Lu L, et al. Using a Fuzzy neural network in clinical decision support for patients with advanced heart failure. IEEE Int Conf Bioinform Biomed 2019;00:995–9.

35. Kwon JM, Kim KH, Jeon KH, et al. Artificial intelligence algorithm for predicting mortality of patients with acute heart failure. PLoS One 2019;14(7): e0219302.

36. Loghmanpour NA, Kormos RL, Kanwar MK, et al. A Bayesian model to predict right ventricular failure following left ventricular assist device therapy. JACC Heart Fail 2016;4(9):711–21.

37. Kanwar MK, Lohmueller LC, Kormos RL, et al. A Bayesian Model to predict survival after left ventricular assist device implantation. JACC Heart Fail 2018;6(9):771–9.

38. Wang Y, Simon MA, Bonde P, et al. Decision tree for adjuvant right ventricular support in patients receiving a left ventricular assist device. J Heart Lung Transplant 2012;31(2):140–9.

39. Movahedi F, Kormos RL, Lohmueller L, et al. Sequential pattern mining of longitudinal adverse events after left ventricular assist device implant. IEEE J Biomed Health 2019;24(8):2347–58.

40. Kilic A, Dochtermann D, Padman R, et al. Using machine learning to improve risk prediction in durable left ventricular assist devices. PLoS One 2021; 16(3):e0247866.

41. Jaeger BC, Cantor RS, Sthanam V, et al. Improving mortality predictions for patients with mechanical circulatory support using follow-up data and machine learning. Circ Genom Precis Med 2020;13(2): e002877.

42. Kilic A, Macickova J, Duan L, et al. Machine learning approaches to analyzing adverse events following durable LVAD implantation. Ann Thorac Surg 2021; 112(3):770–7.

43. Shad R, Quach N, Fong R, et al. Predicting postoperative right ventricular failure using video-based deep learning. Arxiv; 2021.

44. Stöcklmayer C, Dorffner G, Schmidt C, et al. An artificial neural network-based noninvasive detector for suction and left atrium pressure in the control of rotary blood pumps: an in vitro study. Artif Organs 1995;19(7):719–24.

45. Moscato F, Granegger M, Edelmayer M, et al. Continuous monitoring of cardiac rhythms in left ventricular assist device patients. Artif Organs 2014; 38(3):191–8.

46. Mason NO, Bishop CJ, Kfoury AG, et al. Noninvasive predictor of HeartMate XVE pump failure by neural network and waveform analysis. ASAIO J 2010; 56(1):1–5.

47. Hohmann S, Veltmann C, Duncker D, et al. Initial experience with telemonitoring in left ventricular assist device patients. J Thorac Dis 2018;1(1): S853–63.

48. Stehlik J, Schmalfuss C, Bozkurt B, et al. Continuous wearable monitoring analytics predict heart failure hospitalization. Circ Heart Fail 2020;13(3):e006513.

49. Smedira NG, Blackstone EH, Ehrlinger J, et al. Current risks of HeartMate II pump thrombosis: non-parametric analysis of interagency registry for mechanically assisted circulatory support data. J Heart Lung Transpl 2015;34(12):1527–34.

50. Zweck E, Thayer KL, Helgestad OKL, et al. Phenotyping Cardiogenic Shock. J Am Heart Assoc 2020;10(14):e020085.

51. Zhang R, Ma S, Shanahan L, et al. Discovering and identifying New York heart association classification from electronic health records. BMC Med Inform Decis 2018;18(Suppl 2):48.

52. Li Y, Rao S, Solares JRA, et al. BEHRT: transformer for electronic health records. Sci Rep 2020;10(1):7155.

53. Genovese D, Rashedi N, Weinert L, et al. Machine learning–based three-dimensional echocardiographic quantification of right ventricular size and function: validation against cardiac magnetic resonance. J Am Soc Echocardiogr 2019;32(8):969–77.

54. Beecy AN, Bratt A, Yum B, et al. Development of novel machine learning model for right ventricular quantification on echocardiography—a multimodality validation study. Echocardiography 2020;37(5): 688–97.

55. Chen XJ, Collins LM, Patel PA, et al. Heart sound analysis individuals supported with left ventricular assist device: a first look. Comput Cardiol 2020;00:1–4.

56. Misumi Y, Miyagawa S, Yoshioka D, et al. Prediction of aortic valve regurgitation after continuous-flow left ventricular assist device implantation using artificial intelligence trained on acoustic spectra. J Artif Organs 2021;24(2):164–72.

57. Lüneburg N, Reiss N, Feldmann C, et al. Photographic LVAD driveline wound infection recognition using deep learning. Stud Health Technol Inform 2019;260:192–9.

58. Esteva A, Robicquet A, Ramsundar B, et al. A guide to deep learning in healthcare. Nat Med 2019;25(1): 24–9.

59. Rajkomar A, Oren E, Chen K, et al. Scalable and accurate deep learning with electronic health records. NPJ Digit Med 2018;1(1):18.

60. Houser SR. The American Heart Association's New Institute for Precision Cardiovascular Medicine. Circulation 2016;134(24):1913–4.

61. Molina EJ, Shah P, Kiernan MS, et al. The Society of Thoracic Surgeons Intermacs 2020 Annual Report. Ann Thorac Surg 2021;111:778–92.

62. Desai RJ, Wang SV, Vaduganathan M, et al. Comparison of machine learning methods with traditional models for use of administrative claims with electronic medical records to predict heart failure outcomes. JAMA Netw Open 2020;3(1):e1918962.

63. Christodoulou E, Ma J, Collins GS, et al. A systematic review shows no performance benefit of machine learning over logistic regression for clinical prediction models. J Clin Epidemiol 2019;110:12–22.

64. Ginestra JC, Giannini HM, Schweickert WD, et al. Clinician perception of a machine learning–based early warning system designed to predict severe sepsis and septic shock. Crit Care Med 2019; 47(11):1477–84.

65. Lundberg S, Lee SI. A unified approach to interpreting model predictions. Arxiv; 2017.

66. Tseng PY, Chen YT, Wang CH, et al. Prediction of the development of acute kidney injury following cardiac surgery by machine learning. Crit Care 2020;24(1): 478.

67. Bodenheimer T, Sinsky C. From triple to quadruple aim: care of the patient requires care of the provider. Ann Fam Med 2014;12(6):573–6.

68. Kelly CJ, Karthikesalingam A, Suleyman M, et al. Key challenges for delivering clinical impact with artificial intelligence. BMC Med 2019;17(1):195.

Utilizing Conversational Artificial Intelligence, Voice, and Phonocardiography Analytics in Heart Failure Care

Jai Kumar Nahar, MD, MBA[a],*, Francisco Lopez-Jimenez, MD, MS, MBA[b]

KEYWORDS

- Conversational AI • Voice technology • Voice biomarker • Phonocardiography • Heart failure
- Machine learning • Artificial intelligence

KEY POINTS

- Conversational AI agents have great potential to augment and optimize care for heart failure patients.
- Codevelopment of innovative solutions using conversational AI should be undertaken with Multistakeholder collaboration, such as payers, providers, patients, regulators, industry, and academia.
- Phonocardiography is a relatively simple way to assess left ventricular function and is grossly underused in clinical medicine in the United States.
- Machine learning has the potential to increase the diagnostic accuracy of phonocardiography to assess left ventricular function, response to therapy, and to evaluate prognosis.
- Voice can be used as a biomarker in many conditions, including heart failure. Technology is evolving to allow clinicians to diagnose heart failure and to assess prognosis of patients living with heart failure.

INTRODUCTION

The Fourth Industrial Revolution has introduced many important technologies, which are becoming an integral part of our lives. These include voice-powered technologies such as Google Assistant, Alexa, Siri, and Cortana, which are increasingly being used by us in our daily life. Conversational artificial intelligence (CAI) involves the ability of machines (computers, voice-enabled devices) to interact intelligently with the user through the use of voice and voice user interface (VUI). This is made possible by synergistic convergence of voice technology and artificial intelligence (AI) technology[1] (**Fig. 1**).

Why Voice Now? History and Drivers of Adoption

Over the past 4 decades, human-computer interaction has progressed through various stages, as shown in **Fig. 2**, Graphical user interface (GUI), Web interface, Mobile interface, and now Voice user interface (VUI).

With advancements in technology, voice is emerging as an important interface for human-computer interaction. As a result, there is an increase in voice-enabled applications across different sectors of the economy. Health care is an important sector that can leverage voice technology across its different industry verticals, including health care delivery.

[a] Division of Cardiology, Children's National Heart Institute, Children's National Hospital 111 Michigan Avenue, NW, Suite WW3-200 Washington DC, 20010, USA; [b] Department of Cardiovascular Medicine, Mayo Clinic, Mayo Medical School, 200 Second Street, Southwest, Rochester, MN 55901, USA
* Corresponding author.
E-mail address: jnahar@cnmc.org

Heart Failure Clin 18 (2022) 311–323
https://doi.org/10.1016/j.hfc.2021.11.006
1551-7136/22/© 2021 Elsevier Inc. All rights reserved.

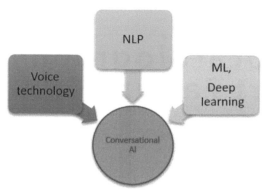

Fig. 1. Conversational AI is made possible by a synergistic convergence of voice technology and artificial intelligence technology (NLP, ML, and deep learning). ML, machine learning; NLP, natural language processing.

There are 3 important reasons why it is an opportune time now for the health care sector to adopt voice technology:

I. Voice is convenient to use because it is the most natural form of human communication. In addition, it offers content, context and rich metadata, and voice biomarkers, which can be used for predictive analytics.

II. Advancements in natural language processing, deep learning, and cloud computing are enabling an increase in the functionality of voice-enabled applications.

III. From the economic perspective, the decrease in price point at which these voice technologies are currently being offered in the market has increased affordability with the potential for widespread adoption.

Outline of This Review

This review article provides an overview and current state of voice technology and CAI and how these can be used for heart failure care delivery. Subsequently, there is a discussion of voice biomarkers and phonocardiography (PCG), and their role in heart failure care (**Fig. 3**).

The review concludes with challenges in the adoption of voice technology, CAI, PCG, and future directions.

DIGITAL VOICE EXPERIENCE, CURRENT STATE: CAI ECOSYSTEM

At present, there are many ways in which we encounter CAI in our daily lives, as mentioned in the following and also illustrated in **Fig. 4**. The components of this ecosystem can be used creatively for heart failure care delivery, per need of the patient.

1. Smart speakers
2. Smart displays, which are the next evolution of smart speakers and include voice technology with touch screen display
3. Smart voice-enabled devices/voice technology integrated digital hubs
4. Two common applications of CAI are virtual assistants and chatbots, these are also known as virtual or conversational agents. A chatbot is a

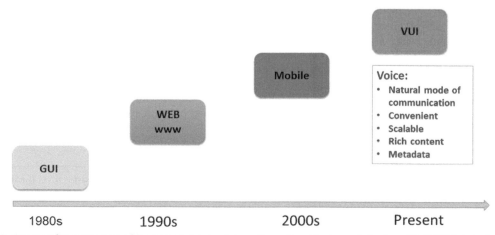

Fig. 2. Stages of progression of human-computer interaction: Graphical user interface (GUI), Web interface, Mobile interface, and now Voice user interface (VUI).

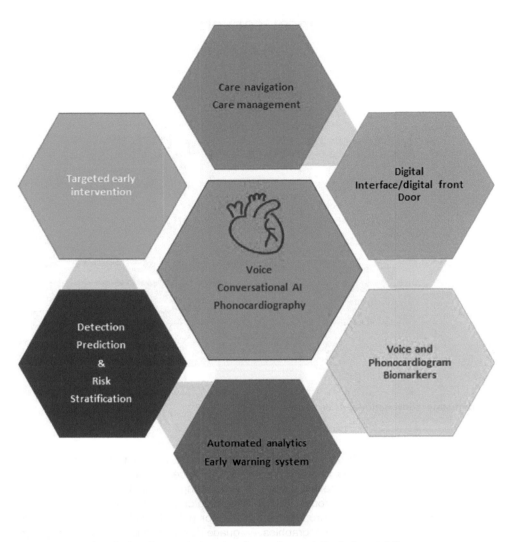

Hexagons contain the following labels:

Care navigation
Care management

Targeted early intervention

Digital Interface/digital front Door

Voice
Conversational AI
Phonocardiography

Detection
Prediction
&
Risk
Stratification

Voice and
Phonocardiogram
Biomarkers

Automated analytics
Early warning system

Fig. 3. Using conversational AI, voice, and phonocardiography analytics in heart failure care.

CAI application that is capable of providing information to the user (patient). A virtual assistant (eg, Apple's Siri, Google Assistant, and Amazon Alexa) is an AI-inspired software agent that is capable of performing certain tasks or services via text or voice.

5. Ambient clinical intelligence is a novel emerging CAI application, which integrates ambient voice sensing and virtual assistant functions.

CLINICAL APPLICATION: VOICE AUGMENTED HEART FAILURE CARE DELIVERY

Among cardiovascular disorders, heart failure is an important cause of morbidity and mortality and contributes to high health care costs. As shown in **Fig. 5** and described in the following, CAI can be leveraged at various stages in heart failure

care delivery, benefiting the patients, providers, and payers, by providing timely access to needed care, filling the gaps in current care model, optimizing management, improving quality of care, and reducing cost.[2,3]

Use of Voice in Outpatient Heart Failure Clinics/Virtual Visits

Electronic Health Records (EHR) documentation and retrieval: CAI-powered voice assistants, which integrate with EHR and virtual visit platforms, can be used at point of care (POC), during in-person clinic visits/virtual visits, by physicians to promptly document information regarding a patient's encounter into the EHR. This enables frictionless, time-efficient documentation, and compliance with coding, billing, and regulatory requirements.

Digital voice experience: conversational AI ecosystem

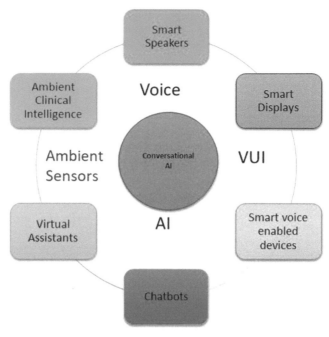

Fig. 4. Current state: conversational AI ecosystem.

The other important function of these virtual voice assistants is to help the physicians to query and retrieve information pertaining to a patient's prior visits, hospitalizations, emergency room visits, labs, imaging studies, interventional procedures, medication refills status, and social/demographics data, from the EHR. By decreasing the nonproductive time that physicians are forced to devote for data input and retrieval from the current EHR systems, voice-assistant integrated smart EHR systems will help to decrease their administrative workload.

Ambient clinical intelligence: This is a novel emerging CAI application, which integrates ambient voice sensing technology and virtual assistant function, to automate and streamline the visit documentation into the EHR, and data retrieval from the EHR by a physician, during a patient's clinic encounter.

Clinical decision support: Voice integrated clinical decision support system can be used by the physicians at the POC to help with diagnosis and planning optimum management of the patient, especially the high-risk patients with multiple comorbidities.

Foreign language interpretation: Access to foreign language interpretation service can be

constrained by cost and geographic location. Smart voice assistants using Natural Language Processing (machine translation) and machine learning can facilitate foreign language interpretation for patients with heart failure who have language barriers and are seen in person in an outpatient clinic or virtually.

Use of Voice at Home

Voice technology used by CAI has an important advantage. It can bypass the traditional mode of human interaction with computers and digital devices, which is through typing and touch screens. Heart failure patients (especially the elderly or visually impaired) who have difficulty interacting with computers through these traditional modes can easily do so now using the currently available intelligent voice technology. CAI-enabled virtual assistants and chatbots can help the patients in promoting wellness and disease management at home. These virtual assistants can help heart failure patients in scheduling and preparing for the upcoming appointments, serve as personal health coach facilitating disease education, chronic care management, treatment adherence, and active engagement in their health care journey. They

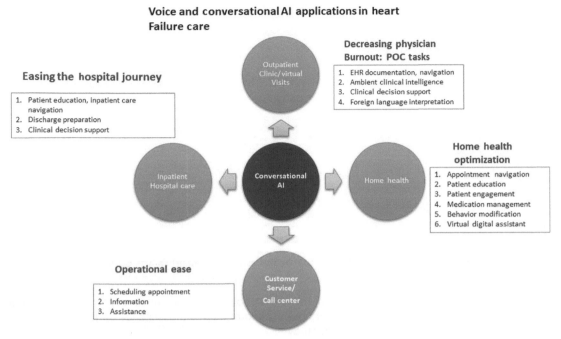

Fig. 5. Important applications of voice technology and conversational AI in heart failure care delivery. POC, point of care.

can offer ongoing personalized care with a touch of empathy, anytime, as needed within the comfort of the patient's own home. By serving as an intelligent digital interface between patients and providers, they can promote 2-way conversation and health information exchange between them as needed.

Fig. 6 illustrates the functional spectrum of voice-enabled virtual health assistant in heart failure care, which includes 3 important functional groups:

- First is to provide assistance to the patients with virtual triage, provide general and specific medical information, assistance with scheduling appointments, prescription refills, connecting with providers, care navigation, and education.
- Second is use as a digital interface (digital front door) between patient and provider, thus helping for home-based remote monitoring, which is evolving as an important component of heart failure care and hospital at home program.
- Third is to work as personal health assistant and wellness coach to enable chronic heart failure care management, including digital therapeutics, behavior modification, and promotion of wellness.

Apergi and colleagues[4] have studied the factors that influence heart failure patients' adoption of voice interface technology used in telehealth. They studied voice technology using 2 different user interfaces, Alexa+ (virtual assistant AI technology developed by Amazon) and a visual Avatar developed by Oben. The authors found that:

1. Black patients used the technology less frequently than other patients with similar characteristics.

2. Patients taking a higher number of medications to manage heart failure interacted less on average with the technology.

3. Older patients tend to exhibit higher levels of engagement with voice interface technologies.

This study indicates that ease of use of voice interface technology in older patients, high disease burden for sicker patients, and social determinants of health in black patients can be the human factors affecting the adoption of voice interface technologies used in a telehealth program for heart failure care delivery.

For patients with heart failure, voice technology–enabled self-care management solutions can be used to optimize their long-term heart failure management. Lee and colleagues conducted a study to evaluate whether a new information communication technology (ICT)–based telehealth program

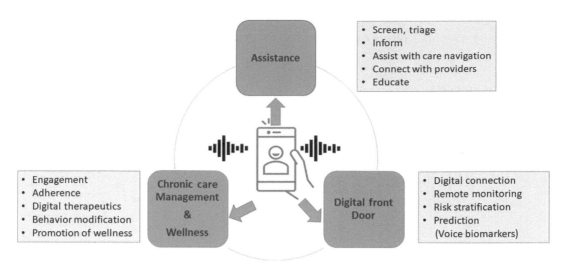

Fig. 6. Functional spectrum of voice-enabled virtual health assistant in heart failure care.

with voice recognition technology could improve clinical or laboratory outcomes in heart failure patients.[5] In this prospective single-arm pilot study comprising 31 patients with chronic heart failure, an ICT-based telehealth program with voice recognition technology was used by patients for 12 weeks. Mobile phone, landline, or the Internet were used to collect patients' comprehensive data elements related to the risk of heart failure self-care management. The study endpoints were the changes observed in urine sodium concentration (uNa), Minnesota Living with Heart Failure (MLHFQ) scores, 6-min walk test, and N-terminal prohormone of brain natriuretic peptide (NT-proBNP) as surrogate markers for appropriate heart failure management.

The study showed that in patients with good adherence to ICT-based telehealth programs, there was a significant improvement in the mean uNa. Similarly, a marginal improvement in MLHFQ scores was only observed in patients with good adherence. The authors concluded that the short-term application of an ICT-based telehealth program with voice recognition technology in heart failure demonstrated the potential to improve control of sodium intake and quality of life in chronic heart failure patients with good adherence to this program. Such programs have the potential to achieve better heart failure care and clinical outcomes.

Use of Voice for Operational Efficiency

Voice-enabled chatbots/virtual agents integrated with institutional Web sites/patient portals can function as virtual call centers/customer service agents and help the patients for automated appointment scheduling, and for providing general information and assistance for the appointments.

Use of Voice in the Hospital

During inpatient hospitalization for heart failure, voice can be used by patients to access information regarding their care team, seek answers to simple questions, search educational content relevant to their hospitalization, and prepare for post-discharge care at home.

VOICE-ENABLED INNOVATION IN HEART FAILURE CARE DELIVERY
Voice-Enabled Heart Failure Care Delivery: Connected Care Model

A challenge for heart failure care is how to achieve comprehensive and continuous care for high-risk patients with multiple comorbidities? How do we complement the current episodic center-based care with optimal remote care and leverage digital health technologies to achieve a hybrid care model which enables comprehensive and continuous care for these patients?

An innovative voice-enabled heart failure care delivery model, as illustrated in **Fig. 7**, can be used to augment and optimize care delivery for these patients improving care access, quality, outcomes, and decrease cost of care. This voice-enabled connected care model has 3 important interconnected components. First is remotely monitored patient and voice-enabled virtual assistant, second is the AI engine, and third is the multi-disciplinary care delivery team. Patient's voice commands and digital remote monitoring signals are transmitted via the virtual voice assistant integrated digital hub/gateway to the AI engine and as

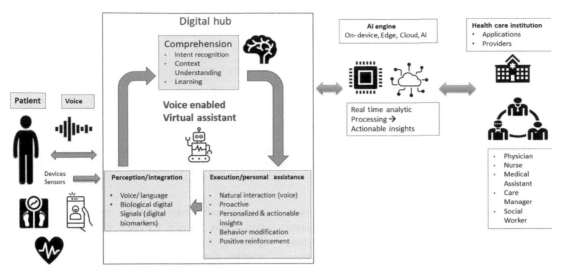

Fig. 7. Innovation in heart failure care delivery: voice-enabled connected care model.

needed to the care delivery team. The AI engine enables real-time analytical processing of this input and in conjunction with the care delivery team, provides personalized and actionable health-promoting insights, delivered back to the patient via voice-enabled virtual assistant. This is a good example of man-machine intelligence synergy and leverages technology such as remote monitoring devices, voice, virtual assistants, AI to connect patients to the care providers, augmenting and optimizing care delivery at home.

VOICE BIOMARKERS AND VOICE ANALYTICS
Voice as A Biomarker in Heart Failure Detection and Management

It is known that different diseases can alter the human voice, either by directly affecting the vocal cords or any of the mechanisms involved in the production of voice such as breathing, expiratory effort, mood, or anatomic changes to the upper airway, including glottis, epiglottis, and tongue. Work on voice as a biomarker has been predominately focused in the field of neurologic degenerative disorders, such as Parkinson disease and Alzheimer disease. Parkinson disease affects phonation and articulation of voice, whereas Alzheimer disease affects verbal fluency, language syntax, and other factors related to the structure of language. Voice as a biomarker has also been tested in other conditions like multiple sclerosis, rheumatoid arthritis, COVID-19 and depression, and other psychiatric conditions.[6–14] In recent years, voice analysis using AI has also been incorporated in the cardiology arena with some landmark publications showing that voice analysis using AI can identify people with coronary disease

or heart failure.[15,16] It is known that heart failure can cause edema of the vocal cord, leading to voice changes. It has also been hypothesized that pulmonary edema affects phonation and speech and respiration.[17] Therefore, it is biologically plausible that heart failure could be diagnosed through voice analysis. The process through which voice is processed and analyzed as a potential biomarker is shown in **Fig. 8**.

Reddy and colleagues have demonstrated that voice analysis using machine learning could identify patients with heart failure. In a study including 20 heart failure patients and 25 healthy controls, the investigators trained a model through feature extraction focused on the glottal features which characterize different aspects of the voice, as well as the mel-frequency cepstral coefficients that mainly captures the vocal tract information of speech (while the glottal features represent the source information of the speech production mechanism). Using support-vector machine (SVM) classifiers and feedforward neural networks and dividing the data sets into training and testing groups, they were able to demonstrate very good accuracy to identify people with heart failure. When creating a speaker-dependent mode model, the classification accuracy reached 95%, whereas speaker-independent mode models achieved a more modest classification accuracy of 81.5%.[15]

In another study, Maor and colleagues demonstrated that voice biomarkers help to discriminate patients with heart failure at low versus high risk for death at follow-up. In this cohort study of more than 10,000 patients who were registered to a call center and had many chronic conditions, including heart failure, the investigators used 223 acoustic features from 20 seconds of recorded

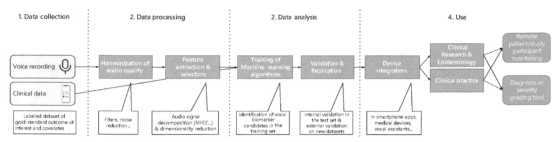

Fig. 8. Pipeline for vocal biomarker identification, from research to practice. (*From* Fagherazzi G, Fischer A, Ismael M, Despotovic V. Voice for Health: The Use of Vocal Biomarkers from Research to Clinical Practice. Digit Biomark. 2021 Apr 16;5(1):78 to 88.; with permission)

speech for each patient. They developed a voice biomarker from a training cohort of nonheart failure patients and then tested it in a cohort of heart failure patients. They extracted low-level acoustic features from each sample using voice processing techniques. The features included speech loudness, jitter, mel cepstrum representation, and shimmer. They then created a machine learning linear model constructed on the training cohort and estimated the hazard ratio of different groups according to the strength of the voice biomarker. They showed that for each standard deviation increase in the biomarker, there was a 32% increased risk of death during follow-up. When comparing the lowest quartile, patients in the top quartile were 96% more likely to die during follow-up. It was remarkable to see that those results were adjusted for known clinical and demographic predictors of mortality.

Those studies show the enormous potential voice analysis has when it comes to identifying patients with heart failure and determining their prognoses. Future studies will need to demonstrate that those results are reproducible and applicable to different settings. Although voice analysis as a biomarker has been shown to be language and accent independent, more data are needed to confirm that many voice features are not influenced by language, accent, and other factors that may theoretically affect the performance of voice as a biomarker in a disease setting.

With the increasing voice data available from the widespread use of voice-enabled smart devices in our daily lives, telephone communications, and emerging ambient voice technology, the potential to use voice as a biomarker to identify and manage heart failure is enormous and scalable.

PCG ANALYTICS IN HEART FAILURE CARE
PCG: Basic Principles

Since the invention of the stethoscope by Rene Laennec in 1816, clinicians have relied on the auscultation of heart sounds to diagnose cardiac conditions. Unfortunately, cardiac auscultation has been shown to lack diagnostic accuracy, given its subjective nature, as shown by multiple studies showing significant disagreement among examiners when interpreting auscultation data.[18,19] In addition to that, the limitations of a human auditory range of sound wavelength is another explanation for the deficiency of physical auscultation.[20] To overcome these limitations, scientists have developed the graphic representation of the sound waves created by heart sounds and murmurs, developing what is now known as PCG. PCG records heart sounds with a microphone attached to the chest wall, and the acoustic signal is then transformed into graphic wavelets that are recorded graphically. The PCG will capture all heart sounds including first sound (S1), second sound (S2), other heart sounds that may represent pathologies like the third and fourth heart sounds, as well as murmurs, snaps, and clicks. Different components of a phonocardiogram are shown in **Fig. 9**.

PCG has been traditionally used to assess physicians' auscultatory skills, but its use has been extended to diagnose cardiac conditions, including left ventricular dysfunction, myocardial ischemia, and valvar heart disease.

PCG Application to Diagnose Heart Failure

The analysis of heart sounds through PCG has shown a good correlation with different measures of left ventricular systolic function. The most common parameter has been the systolic time interval, defined as the interval between the peak intensity of the S1 and S2.[21,22] Overtime, the PCG has been combined with electrocardiography (ECG) signals leading to better accuracy to detect left ventricular dysfunction. The study by Stack and colleagues demonstrated that pre-ejection time divided by ejection time combining ECG and PCG signals yielded a sensitivity of 88% and a specificity of 96% to detect left ventricular systolic dysfunction with an excellent interobserver agreement.[23] Other

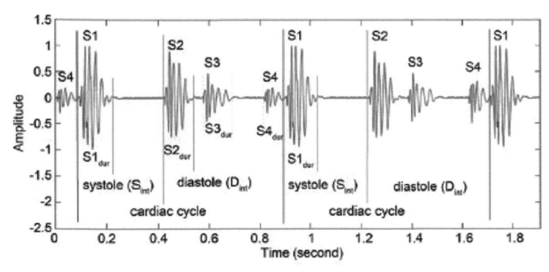

Fig. 9. Different components of a phonocardiogram, including cardiac sounds first (S1), second (S2), third (S3), and fourth (S4). (*From* Nabih-Ali M, El-Dahshan EA, Yahia AS. A review of intelligent systems for heart sound signal analysis. J Med Eng Technol. 2017 Oct;41(7):553-563; *with permission.*)

studies have shown that PCG in combination with ECG signals can detect left ventricular dysfunction as precisely as echocardiographic parameters, including left ventricular ejection fraction.[24–26] In one study with 161 patients with heart failure, the authors demonstrated that several PCG parameters had excellent concordance with echocardiography-measured left ventricular ejection fraction.[24] Other studies have shown that PCG can predict low left ventricular ejection fraction more accurately than BNP.[25] Studies measuring left ventricular systolic function invasively by determining the left ventricular dp/dt and pulmonary capillary wedge pressure have demonstrated that PCG could predict well left ventricular dysfunction.[27] More recent studies have shown that PCG in combination with ECG signals can discriminate between heart failure with preserved ejection fraction from heart failure with reduced ejection fraction, with an area under the ROC curve of 0.81, a sensitivity of 53%, and a specificity of 91%. Those values had a similar diagnostic performance that echocardiographic measures of left ventricular restrictive patterns such as mitral annulus tissue velocity, to differentiate heart failure with preserved ejection fraction from heart failure with reduced ejection fraction.[28] In the same study, investigators also demonstrated similar diagnostic performance using PCG to differentiate cardiac versus noncardiac causes of dyspnea. More recent studies have assessed the value of PCG to monitor left ventricular function in cancer patients receiving cardiotoxic drugs. In a prospective study including 187 patients treated with anthracyclines, parameters

extracted from PCG showed a sensitivity of 88% and a specificity of 84% to identify left ventricular systolic dysfunction confirmed by echocardiography.[29]

The parameters derived from PCG in conjunction with ECG signals include the electromechanical activation time (EMAT), which represents the time required to generate force by the left ventricle to close the mitral valve and is therefore related to how quickly the left ventricle generates pressure. Other parameters include the percent EMAT, which is the ratio of EMAT to the RR interval, the left ventricular systolic time or time between S1 and S2, and the presence and strength of third and fourth cardiac sounds, among other parameters.[30]

PCG has several limitations as it relies on the quality of the recording of the cardiac sounds; therefore, endogenous and exogenous noises will affect the diagnostic accuracy and the interpretation of the PCG. Other limitations include the difficulty to determine the exact onset, peak, and end of cardiac sounds in the PCG, variability of sound intensity across subjects, and the challenges to perform PCG in patients with heart failure who may not be able to hold their breath or to lay flat on the examination bed.

Incorporation of Machine Learning to Interpret PCG

In recent years, investigators have been working on using machine learning techniques in the interpretation of the PCG to create automatic analysis and reporting, and to potentially tap into

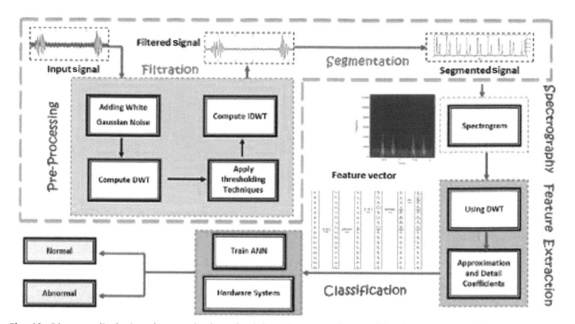

Fig. 10. Diagram displaying the standard methodology incorporating machine learning to evaluate PCG. (*From* Nabih-Ali M, El-Dahshan EA, Yahia AS. A review of intelligent systems for heart sound signal analysis. J Med Eng Technol. 2017 Oct;41(7):553-563; with permission.)

diagnostic capabilities that go beyond the traditional interpretation of PCG signals.

The drawbacks of PCG include the inability to differentiate between separate frequencies of various sounds, the failure to show frequency components information of PCG signals, the frequent presence of noises and artifacts that may visually mask weak heart sounds, and the problem to identify the boundaries of heart sounds. In principle, machine learning could help overcome those technical challenges.

The architecture of machine learning–based models to interpret PCG signals requires several key steps, as shown in **Fig. 10**. First, PCG signals need to be preprocessed to create cleaner soundwave signals. This is generally carried out through several steps, including filtering the signals using high-pass filters to remove unwanted low-frequency signals; white denoising, where PCG signals are filtered to remove white noise using wavelet packet; and finally through normalization, where the PCG signals are normalized to the expected amplitude of the signal.

The second stage in the preprocessing of PCG signals involves signal segmentation. During this phase, the computer learns to identify the different soundwave components of the cardiac cycle and to identify abnormal sounds and murmurs. Once the preprocessing is completed, the next step is feature extraction and classification of the PCG signals. There are many techniques used to carry out feature extraction of PCG signals, including

linear frequency band cepstral, discrete cosine transformation, Fourier transformation, and others. The classification stage is generally carried out through one or more approaches, including neural networks, SVMs, self-organizing maps, and hybrid techniques. At this stage, the investigators need to define the labels to train the algorithm in which the purpose of the algorithm is established whether it is to identify normal patterns, to detect specific cardiac conditions, or to aid in the determination of prognosis. More recently, investigators have used recurrent neural networks to obviate feature extraction to make the PCG processing more efficient, with accuracies that were as good as or better than other models requiring feature extraction.[31]

PCG Analysis Using AI to Diagnose Heart Failure

Although PCG analysis to diagnose left ventricular systolic dysfunction has been extensively investigated using traditional statistical techniques, the potential of machine learning application to PCG to diagnose heart failure remains in its infancy. In one study by Gao and colleagues, they were able to identify heart failure using adversarial neural networks to assess PCG signals, with an outstanding diagnostic accuracy of 98.8%.[31] In that study, the investigators were not only able to identify heart failure but also to differentiate heart failure with preserved ejection fraction versus

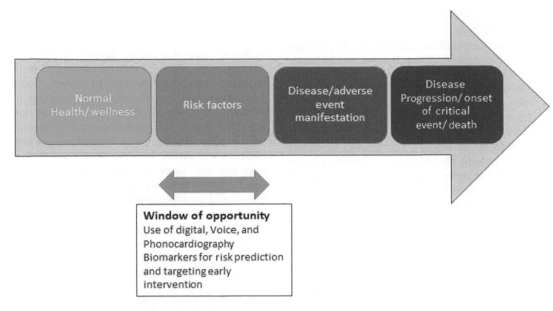

Fig. 11. Timeline of disease progression for heart failure patients and window of opportunity.

heart failure with reduced ejection fraction in 108 heart failure patients and 1297 healthy subjects and more than 7600 PCG signals. If confirmed in other studies and other patient settings, those results show the immense potential of PCG-AI (PCG integrated with AI) to identify people with heart failure and open new avenues for comparisons against other biomarkers and clinical decision rules used to diagnose heart failure.

Summary of the Evidence Using AI to Interpret PCG Signals to Diagnose Heart Failure

Although data evaluating the value of AI in the interpretation of PCG signals is very preliminary, early results are very promising, underscoring the huge potential of AI to offer automated analytics and intelligent insights from PCG. Future studies are needed to apply these principles to clinically validated data sets to determine the real-life diagnostic accuracy of PCG to diagnose heart failure, to differentiate heart failure with preserved versus decreased ejection fraction, and to determine the prognostic value of AI-based PCG analysis among patients with heart failure. Other future potential applications include the evaluation of therapeutic response to guideline-based medical therapies or monitoring the improvement or deterioration of left ventricular systolic function over time.

Early Warning Systems: Using Voice and PCG Biomarkers in Heart Failure Care

As shown in **Fig. 11**, in the timeline of heart failure progression, there is a window of opportunity

where innovative digital biomarkers (such as voice biomarkers and PCG biomarkers) can be incorporated in specially designed intelligent early warning systems, helping in prompt identification of at-risk patients and targeting timely appropriate therapeutic interventions. This will be very helpful to prevent adverse outcomes due to heart failure progression and its associated morbidity and mortality.

CHALLENGES IN THE ADOPTION OF VOICE TECHNOLOGY, CAI, AND PCG

As we look forward to scaling and widespread adoption of voice technology, CAI, and PCG in heart failure care, the following challenges need to be considered:

- *Data Sharing*: Sharing of curated and deidentified databases integrating voice and PCG biomarkers is a great challenge, but an important step for advancing future research, development of sound evidence, and optimal clinical integration for augmenting heart failure care.
- *Privacy and Security*: Maintenance of privacy and security of health information is integral to ensure against unauthorized access and misuse of personal health information.
- *Accuracy*: To obtain proper results from the use of CAI system, the human voice has to be accurately comprehended by the voice-enabled devices and with minimal noise. Failure to do so will result in inefficient use and

patient frustration and erroneous signals and interpretations.

- *Optimal Design/User Experience*: The design of these voice-enabled devices should facilitate their smooth and painless integration in the daily life routine of the patients, especially old patients who may not be technology savvy.
- *Reliability and Trust:* The content, which is generated by the CAI system and delivered to the patient, should be from a reliable source and trustworthy. PCG and voice as a biomarker need to prove in future studies the accuracy of the PCG and voice signals to diagnose heart failure and other cardiac conditions and to assess prognosis. They also need to prove added value on top and above current technology.
- *Ethics*: Data from CAI systems should not be unethically used to the disadvantage of the patients. Implementation of systems using CAI or voice as a biomarker needs to keep confidentiality and respect privacy.
- *Reimbursement:* There should be buy-in from the payers, so the reimbursement for this technology is not a barrier in its widespread adoption.

FUTURE DIRECTIONS

Looking ahead in the future, consideration should be given to humanizing these digital CAI agents by making their response proactive, incorporating context-specific empathy for the patients, developing cognitive capabilities for them, and incorporating on-device AI, so they can be great companions and assets for the heart failure patients.

In regards to PCG, clinical trials incorporating AI in the processing of PCG signals will help to define the clinical utility when applied to real-life scenarios. They may help to screen for individuals with systolic or diastolic left ventricular dysfunction, to better define the prognosis of patients with heart failure, and certainly to expand its diagnostic and prognostic capabilities beyond heart failure.

Studies using voice as a biomarker to diagnose heart failure or to assess its prognosis need to be conducted in different languages, testing the effect of accents, variations during conversational voice, and other potential sources of error, to better understand the reproducibility of this signal as a biomarker. Ethical issues including confidentiality need to be considered when implementing systems using voice as a biomarker to diagnose cardiac and other medical conditions.

SUMMARY

CAI agents have great potential to augment and optimize care for heart failure patients. For maximum benefit from this technology, we need to incorporate design thinking to deliver good patient experience and smooth, pain-free integration in their daily routine. Codevelopment of innovative solutions should be undertaken with multistakeholder collaboration, such as payers, providers, patients, regulators, industry, and academia. Privacy and security of data and promotion of ethical use for the benefit of patients are integral to their successful implementation.

Early warning systems, which use digital voice and PCG biomarkers for heart failure care, have great potential in prompt identification of at-risk patients and targeting timely appropriate interventions.

CAI, voice technology, voice and PCG analytics, is an emerging frontier in health care and has great potential to bring digital transformation of heart failure care delivery.

CLINICS CARE POINTS

- Although data evaluating the value of artificial intelligence (AI) in the interpretation of phonocardiography (PCG) signals is very preliminary, early results are very promising, underscoring the enormous potential of AI to offer automated analytics and intelligent insights from PCG.
- Early warning systems, which use digital voice and PCG biomarkers for heart failure, have great potential in prompt identification of at-risk patients and targeting timely appropriate interventions. Research is needed to validate the utility of voice and PCG biomarkers in clinical practice.
- Conversational AI agents have great potential to augment and optimize care for heart failure patients. Pilot studies to evaluate their efficacy, followed by multistakeholder collaboration to codesign innovative solutions and sharing of best practices, will help in the development of evidence and their subsequent integration in clinical practice in the long run.

DISCLOSURE

The authors have nothing to disclose.

REFERENCES

1.. Chang A. Intelligence-based medicine: artificial intelligence and human cognition in clinical medicine and Healthcare. London, United Kingdom: Academic Press; 2020.

2.. Metcalf DS, Fisher T, Pruthi S, et al. Voice technology in Healthcare: Leveraging voice to Enhance patient and provider experiences. Boca Raton, Florida: CRC Press; 2020.

3. Nahar J. Innovation at ACC | Potential of Voice/ Conversational AI in Medicine. In. Cardiology Magazine 2019. Available at: https://bluetoad.com/publication/?m=14537&i=629407&p=1&ver=html5.

4.. Apergi LA, Bjarnadottir MV, Baras JS, et al. Voice interface technology adoption by patients with heart failure: pilot study, 2021 comparison study. JMIR Mhealth Uhealth 2021;9(4):e24646.

5.. Lee H, Park JB, Choi SW, et al. Impact of a telehealth program with voice recognition technology in patients with chronic heart failure: feasibility study. JMIR Mhealth Uhealth 2017;5(10):e127.

6. Fagherazzi G, Fischer A, Ismael M, et al. Voice for Health: The Use of Vocal Biomarkers from Research to Clinical Practice. Digital Biomarkers 2021;5(1): 78–88.

7. Dashtipour K, Tafreshi A, Lee J, et al. Speech disorders in Parkinson's disease: pathophysiology, medical management and surgical approaches. Neurodegener Dis Manag 2018;8(5):337–48.

8. Rudzicz F. Articulatory Knowledge in the Recognition of Dysarthric Speech. IEEE Trans Audio, Speech, Lang Process 2011;19(4):947–60.

9. Toth L, Hoffmann I, Gosztolya G, et al. A Speech Recognition-based Solution for the Automatic Detection of Mild Cognitive Impairment from Spontaneous Speech. Curr Alzheimer Res 2018;15(2):130–8.

10. Pützer M, Wokurek W, Moringlane JR. Evaluation of Phonatory Behavior and Voice Quality in Patients with Multiple Sclerosis Treated with Deep Brain Stimulation. J Voice 2017;31(4):483–9.

11. Kosztyła-Hojna B, Moskal D, Kuryliszyn-Moskal A. Parameters of the assessment of voice quality and clinical manifestation of rheumatoid arthritis. Adv Med Sci 2015;60(2):321–8.

12. Taguchi T, Tachikawa H, Nemoto K, et al. Major depressive disorder discrimination using vocal acoustic features. J Affect Disord 2018;225:214–20.

13. Cohen AS, Elvevåg B. Automated computerized analysis of speech in psychiatric disorders. Curr Opin Psychiatry 2014;27(3):203–9.

14. Anthes E. Alexa, do I have COVID-19? Nature 2020; 586(7827):22–5.

15. Kiran Reddy M, Helkkula P, Madhu Keerthana Y, et al. The automatic detection of heart failure using speech signals. Computer Speech Lang 2021;69:101205.

16. Maor E, Sara JD, Orbelo DM, et al. Voice Signal Characteristics Are Independently Associated With Coronary Artery Disease. Mayo Clin Proc 2018;93(7):840–7.

17. Murton OM, Hillman RE, Mehta DD, et al. Acoustic speech analysis of patients with decompensated heart failure: A pilot study. The J Acoust Soc America 2017;142(4):EL401–7.

18. Marcus G, Vessey J, Jordan MV, et al. Relationship Between Accurate Auscultation of a Clinically Useful Third Heart Sound and Level of Experience. Arch Intern Med 2006;166(6):617–22.

19. Ishmail AA, Wing S, Ferguson J, et al. Interobserver Agreement by Auscultation in the Presence of a Third Heart Sound in Patients with Congestive Heart Failure. Chest 1987;91(6):870–3.

20. Avendano-Valencia LD, Ferrero JM, Castellanos-Dominguez G. Improved parametric estimation of time frequency representations for cardiac murmur discrimination. Paper presented at: 2008 Computers in Cardiology: Bologna, Italy; September 14–17, 2008, 2008.

21. Garrard CL Jr, Weissler AM, Dodge HT. The relationship of alterations in systolic time intervals to ejection fraction in patients with cardiac disease. Circulation 1970;42(3):455–62.

22. Lewis RP, Rittogers SE, Froester WF, et al. A critical review of the systolic time intervals. Circulation 1977; 56(2):146–58.

23. Weissler AM, Harris WS, Schoenfeld CD. Bedside technics for the evaluation of ventricular function in man. Am J Cardiol 1969;23(4):577–83.

24. Zuber M, Kipfer P, Attenhofer Jost C. Systolic dysfunction: correlation of acoustic cardiography with Doppler echocardiography. Congest Heart Fail 2006;12(Suppl 1):14–8.

25. Kosmicki DL, Collins SP, Kontos MC, et al. Noninvasive prediction of left ventricular systolic dysfunction in patients with clinically suspected heart failure using acoustic cardiography. Congest Heart Fail 2010; 16(6):249–53.

26. Collins SP, Lindsell CJ, Kontos MC, et al. Bedside prediction of increased filling pressure using acoustic electrocardiography. Am J Emerg Med 2009; 27(4):397–408.

27. Collins SP, Kontos MC, Michaels AD, et al. Utility of a bedside acoustic cardiographic model to predict elevated left ventricular filling pressure. Emerg Med J 2010;27(9):677–82.

28. Wang S, Lam Y-Y, Liu M, et al. Acoustic cardiography helps to identify heart failure and its phenotypes. Int J Cardiol 2013;167(3):681–6.

29. Toggweiler S, Odermatt Y, Brauchlin A, et al. The Clinical Value of Echocardiography and Acoustic Cardiography to Monitor Patients Undergoing Anthracycline Chemotherapy. Clin Cardiol 2013;36(4):201–6.

30. Wen YN, Lee AP, Fang F, et al. Beyond auscultation: acoustic cardiography in clinical practice. Int J Cardiol 2014;172(3):548–60.

31. Gao S, Zheng Y, Guo X. Gated recurrent unit-based heart sound analysis for heart failure screening. Biomed Eng Online 2020;19(1):3.

Application of 3D Printing Technology in Heart Failure

Kanwal M. Farooqi, MD[a],*, Jennifer Smerling, MD[a], Ulrich P. Jorde, MD[b]

KEYWORDS

• Heart failure • 3D printing • 3D modeling • Medical modeling • Procedural planning

KEY POINTS

• Optimization of care for patients with heart failure includes the use of advanced imaging.
• 3D imaging datasets can be translated into 3D digital models that can be 3D printed.
• 3D printing allows improved visualization of complex anatomic cardiac structures.
• 3D printed models can aid in preprocedural planning for a wide range of intervention for patients with heart failure.

INTRODUCTION

Heart failure (HF) represents a wide spectrum of disease, defined as impaired ventricular filling or ejection and diagnosed clinically based on symptoms and physical examination. It has an incidence of greater than 650,000 new cases diagnosed yearly in the United States (US).[1] The lifetime risk of HF in Americans older than 40 years of age is 20%, and that incidence only increases with age, costing 1% to 2% of the total health care budget in the US.[1,2] More importantly, absolute mortality for those diagnosed with HF is 50% within 5 years. While potential etiologies of HF are broad and multifactorial, frequent assessment and therapy optimization are crucial for improving long-term outcomes.[2] Current standard of care involves routine imaging with frequent echocardiograms and X-rays as well as the utilization of further advanced imaging modalities when necessary. With the advancement of imaging technology, 3 dimensional (3D) printing has allowed providers to create patient specific, anatomic models for use across multiple medical disciplines.[3] This technology is especially applicable with the rapid increase of novel percutaneous devices coming into use for transcatheter interventions. The goal of this review is to discuss 3D printing as a unique tool for continued evaluation, monitoring, and further intervention for this specific patient population.

3D PRINTED MODEL CREATION

The source images for a 3D printed model can be from a 3D imaging dataset including echocardiogram, cardiac magnetic resonance imaging (MRI), or cardiac computed tomography (CT) dataset. Ideally, there is good blood pool to myocardial contrast in the chosen images. If for example, the blood pool in a set of 3D cardiac MRI images is uniform in its gray values across all planes and is well-differentiated from the myocardium, this will lead to the most straightforward postprocessing. Thresholding, the process by which a range of gray values is specified as the area of interest, becomes much faster and simpler with such a set of images. One specific range will clearly highlight the blood pool but not the myocardium and vice versa. Once the area of interest is highlighted,

[a] Department of Pediatrics, Division of Cardiology, Columbia University Irving Medical Center, New York, NY, USA; [b] Department of Internal Medicine, Division of Cardiology, Montefiore Medical Center, Albert Einstein College of Medicine, Bronx, NY, USA
* Corresponding author. Columbia University Irving Medical Center, 3959 Broadway, CH-2N, New York, NY 10032.
E-mail address: kf2549@cumc.columbia.edu

Heart Failure Clin 18 (2022) 325–333
https://doi.org/10.1016/j.hfc.2021.11.002
1551-7136/22/© 2021 Elsevier Inc. All rights reserved.

the image processing software will create a 3D digital structure based on our specified area of interest. If the blood pool was segmented, another step of creating an external layer and then hollowing this structure is needed to create a "shell" of the blood pool which then represents the intracardiac anatomy. Once a virtual model has been created which is acceptable in quality, it is saved in a standard 3D file format, such as.stl or stereolithography. This can then be printed on a 3D printer to create a physical cardiac replica that can be used for educational or presurgical planning purposes. 3D printers vary in their capabilities in regards to printing "resolution" or layer thickness, printing material and color, build size, and speed. More costly 3D printing systems typically allow a wide variety of options for multi-material and multicolor printing.

SURGICAL PLANNING

One of the most common uses of 3D printed models is preoperative planning for surgical interventions. Surgeons typically use 2 dimensional (2D) representations of 3D anatomic structures to become familiar with a patients' cardiac anatomy. Unique models derived from individual patient's imaging datasets provide both providers and surgeons with accurate, tactile structures in true 3D that they can visualize before entering the OR. This allows them the insight to create unique, patient specific, operative plans. Common uses of 3D cardiac models for presurgical planning include the resection of excess myocardium in hypertrophic cardiomyopathy (HOCM), VAD placement, and modeling for congenital heart disease (CHD).[4–7]

HYPERTROPHIC CARDIOMYOPATHY

For patients with HOCM, 3D printed models have been used for patient education as well as preoperative surgical review. In a study published by Guo and colleagues, 3D models were created for patients with HOCM from their preoperative CT scans for use in discussion between surgeon and patient at their preoperative visit.[8] They found the models to be useful for their understanding of the underlying disease process, as well as the surgical plan. Modeling has also been demonstrated to be helpful specifically to plan the surgical approach. Resection of the interventricular septum is not a very commonly performed procedure. Surgeons must be careful to remove enough tissue to prevent recurrence, occurring in approximately 20% of cases, and yet prudent not to remove too much leading to damage of surrounding tissue.[9]

In a proof-of-concept study, Hermsen and colleagues used 3D printed models for patient-specific planning and operative rehearsal for surgical myectomy of the left ventricular outflow tract (LVOT) in 2 patients with HOCM.[10] Preoperatively patients underwent CT scan with subsequent 3D printing of their hearts. On the day before surgery, the surgeon performed a myectomy on the model in simulated OR conditions. While the utility of these models for HOCM resection must be further validated in larger studies with more quantitative measures, Guo and colleagues were able to demonstrate that they could use the volume of tissue resected on the model to plan the extent of actual tissue resection.[8] Andrushchuk and colleagues took this one step further, by creating 3D models preoperatively and printing "ideal" models after virtual septal myectomy.[4] These models were sterilized and present in the operating room during surgery. The surgeons could then resect mapped sections of the septum and successively fill the surgical zones on the sterilized model until the preplanned volume was approximated. In this way, they were able to improve outcomes and increase the average resected myocardial mass without complications.

VENTRICULAR ASSIST DEVICE PLACEMENT

3D printed models have been useful in the placement of ventricular assist devices (VAD) in adults with CHD. Complex CHD requires a thorough understanding of anatomic relationships in 3D to understand the underlying pathophysiology of each patient.[6] Patient anatomy is often unique and specific, requiring the provider to translate 2D images seen on echo and catheterization into 3D mental representations. The use of 3D models allows providers to better understand anatomy and describe it to both patients and other medical team members in a more straightforward manner. They have been used for patient education, medical education, as well as presurgical planning in this context.[5,11–13] Due to the inherent nature of the disease, many CHD lesions are generally repaired in childhood. As surgical outcomes and overall medical care continue to improve, far more patients with CHD are reaching adulthood than ever before, presenting an evolving challenge for ACHD providers.[14] 3D printed cardiac models serve as a valuable tool to aid in VAD placement in adults with CHD. In a paper previously published by our group, we described the use of 3D printing for preoperative VAD planning in adults with systemic right ventricles and single ventricle circulations.[6] We described how preoperative CT scans were used to create individualized 3D printed

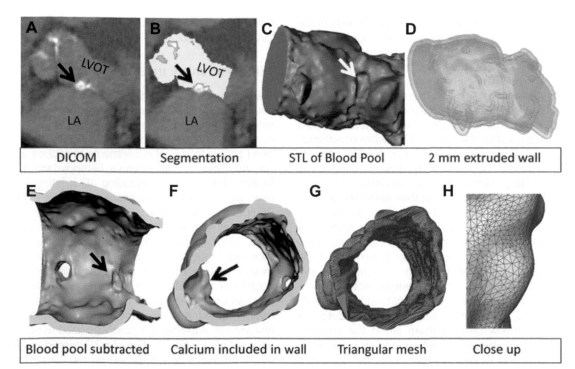

Fig. 1. Creation of a 3D Print of the Left Ventricular Outflow Tract (*A*) Images from a CT dataset of the left ventricular outflow tract (LVOT) demonstrate calcification (*black arrow*). (*B*) Segmentation allows highlighting of the area of interest, in this case, the blood pool of the LVOT. (*C*) The segmentation of the blood pool is translated into a 3 dimensional STL file. (*D*). A 2 mm wall is extruded outward from the 3D STL file to create a hollow structure. (*E, F*). Once the blood pool is subtracted, the calcification is represented (*black arrow*). (*G, H*) The 3D object is comprised of a triangular mesh. (*From* Ripley B, Kelil T, Cheezum MK, Goncalves A, Di Carli MF, Rybicki FJ, Steigner M, Mitsouras D, Blankstein R. 3D printing based on cardiac CT assists anatomic visualization prior to transcatheter aortic valve replacement. J Cardiovasc Comput Tomogr. 2016 Jan-Feb;10(1):28-36; *with permission.*)

models to help guide VAD cannula placement. One of our patients had undergone Mustard procedure for the d-transposition of the great arteries (TGA) in childhood, and the second patient had unrepaired I-TGA and presented in right HF, both required placement of an RVAD. The third patient was a patient with d-TGA who had undergone a Fontan procedure who required systemic ventricular support. A similar process was demonstrated by Miller and colleagues who used 3D printing for a d-TGA patient who had undergone a Mustard procedure.[7] In all cases, surgeons found the models to be helpful in both surgical planning and simulation. While the creation of 3D models is often time-consuming and labor-intensive, they provide surgeons with a more complete understanding of complex anatomy to help plan for surgical procedures and possibly, improve outcomes.

TRANSCATHETER INTERVENTIONS

3D printed models can also aid in the planning of catheter-based interventions, including valve replacements. Unlike their surgical colleagues, interventional cardiologists do not directly visualize

cardiac structures. Instead, they rely on 2D fluoroscopy in multiple views to estimate the size and dimension of cardiac structures during the procedure. This provides a unique dilemma when it comes to device implantation. Interventionalists must estimate the size of the site of implantation and optimize device orientation to minimize the paravalvular leak inherent in a sutureless valve replacement. Direct visualization of the valve annulus using a 3D printed model, allows for a better approximation of the appropriate device size and position.[15]

TRANSCATHETER AORTIC VALVE REPLACEMENT

Ripley and colleagues, assessed patients who had undergone transcatheter aortic valve replacements (TAVRs) who had a preprocedural electrocardiogram gated cardiac CT as well as a postprocedure echocardiogram.[16] (**Fig. 1**) They retrospectively reviewed each patient and created 3D printed models from their preprocedural cardiac CT scans. Researchers found that patient-specific anatomy remained preserved in the 3D representations, and measurements of the annulus and LVOT dimensions, correlated to measurements taken on 2D echocardiogram. In regards to paravalvular aortic regurgitation (PAR); however, they found their predictions to be suboptimal. This was thought to be multifactorial but likely related to the inelastic material used for the 3D printed cardiac model, and the rigid plastic used for the model of the valve prosthesis. Qian and colleagues, however, took a different approach.[17] In their study they retrospectively analyzed patients with varying amounts of PAR and created 3D models of their aortic roots using pre-TAVR cardiac CT imaging. Researchers embedded sinusoidal fibers into the aortic wall models to better approximate the physical properties of human aortic tissue. A series of radiopaque beads were then attached to the outside of the phantom to help detect and measure circumferential strain distribution. Specifically, a bulge index was created to detect a low–high–low strain pattern along the annulus. In this way, the same self-expanding valve prosthesis used in each patient could be implanted in their 3D printed aortic root and a bulge index could be calculated. While they found annular calcification to be the best predictor of moderate–severe PAR after initial placement of the valve, bulge index was a significant predictor of moderate–severe PAR after initial placement, and the only significant predictor postballoon expansion. They demonstrated that not only could human tissue be approximated through the use of 3D printed models but also that models could be used as a quantitative measure for the disease process.

TRANSCATHETER MITRAL VALVE REPLACEMENT

Neo-LVOT obstruction is a significant cause of morbidity and mortality after transcatheter mitral valve replacement. In a prospective study looking at transcatheter mitral valve replacement, Wang and colleagues found that the 3D printed LVOT models were "indispensable tools" for predicting neo-LVOT obstruction.[18,19] Their study used cardiac CT-based computer-aided design and 3D printing of the LVOT to model transcatheter valve size and orientation in the mitral position to help with preprocedural planning. Postprocedural CT scans were then obtained measuring true postprocedural LVOT and compared with model predictions. They found that their models were reproducible and highly predictive of LVOT anatomy. A predicted neo-LVOT ≤ 189.4 mm^2 had 100% sensitivity and 96.8% specificity for Mitral

Valve Academic Research Consortium defined LVOT obstruction.

TRICUSPID VALVE INTERVENTION

Transcatheter caval valve placement has been suggested to treat patients with severe tricuspid valve regurgitation, at risk for right HF, who is not candidates for surgical repair. Such valves have been shown in animal experiments to reduce valvar insufficiency and improve hemodynamics.[20] Multimodality imaging including 3D printing was used by O'Neill and colleagues to implant a SAPIEN XT valve (Edwards Lifesciences Corp., Irvine, California) at the right atrium (RA)–inferior vena cava (IVC) junction in a patient with severe tricuspid regurgitation and decreased right ventricular systolic function. The patient was status postmitral ring placement for mitral regurgitation, had undergone radiation therapy for lymphoma treatment, and had developed significant abdominal ascites. A cardiac CT scan was used to obtain source data for the creation of a 3D printed model of the RA-IVC junction. Based on the 3D printed model, the decision was made to use the SAPIEN 29XT valve as opposed to the SAPIEN 26T valve which demonstrated gaps between the IVC and valve frame concerning sites of possible paravalvular leak. The patient was discharged after 1 week without the recurrence of ascites at 4-month follow-up.[21] Spring and colleagues used a 3D printed cardiac model created from a cardiac CT source dataset to guide valve in the valve replacement of a tricuspid valve with a SAPIEN XT valve in a 44-year high-risk patient with a complex medical history including prior bioprosthetic tricuspid and mechanical mitral valve replacements. There was evidence of severe tricuspid stenosis and fibrosis of the tricuspid valve leaflets. Given the complexity of the anatomy of the region, imaging data were used to recreate a digital and subsequently a 3D print of the right heart (**Fig. 2**). This model was used to simulate the transcatheter approach via the inferior and superior vena cava and a 23 mm balloon-expandable Sapien XT valve (Edwards Lifesciences, Irvine, CA). Based on the information gained from the 3D printed model, a transfemoral approach was used. The digital model was overlain on the fluoroscopy during the procedure, which was completed successfully without complications.[22] In cases in which a MitraClip is being placed in the tricuspid position, 3D printed models have been found to allow the determination of the precise location of the landing zone before the actual intervention. Vukicevic and colleagues reported on this application in 3 patients with severe tricuspid regurgitation in whom the models

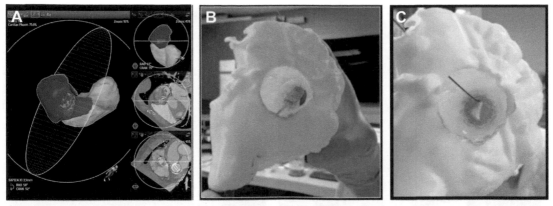

Fig. 2. 3D Printing for the planning of tricuspid valve intervention (*A*) Segmentation of the right atrium (*red*) and ventricle (*green*) to allow estimation of proper valve size. (*B,C*) The 3D digital file was then printed to create a patient-specific model. The model was used to simulate the delivery system with the placement of the 23 mm SAPIEN XT valve. (*From* Spring AM, Pirelli L, Basman CL, Kliger CA. The Importance of Pre-Operative Imaging and 3-D Printing in Transcatheter Tricuspid Valve-in-Valve Replacement. Cardiovasc Revasc Med. 2021 Jul;28S:161-165; *with permission.*)

allowed from the comprehensive assessment of tricuspid valve anatomy as well as the consideration of a more lateral or medial valve position (**Fig. 3**). In one patient, a MitraClip deployment was not undertaken after simulation with the 3D printed model revealed that the coaptation defect remained too large in all configurations of a Mitra-Clip deployment.[23]

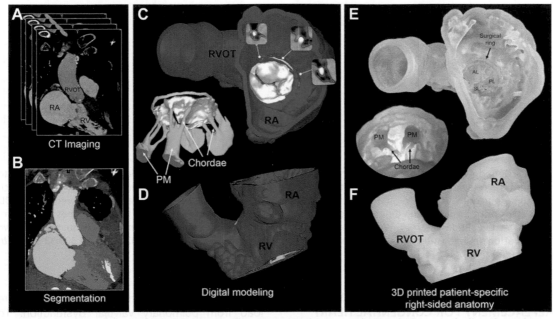

Fig. 3. 3D Printing of the Right Ventricular Outflow Tract (*A, B*) Images of the right heart including the right ventricular outflow tract (RVOT) and tricuspid valve (TV) from cardiac computed tomography (CT) allow for segmentation of the region of interest for digital model creation. (*C*) The right atrium (RA), TV, and RVOT are well represented in the digital reconstruction created from the segmentation of the CT images. (*D*) The chordae and papillary muscles (PM) of the TV were also recreated. (*E, F*) The 3 dimensional (3D) print of the right heart including detailed anatomy of the tricuspid valve. AL, Anterior leaflet; PL, posterior leaflet; PM, papillary muscles; RA, right atrium; RV, right ventricle; RVOT, right ventricle outflow tract; SL, septal leaflet. (*From* Vukicevic M, Faza NN, Avenatti E, Durai PC, El-Tallawi KC, Filippini S, Chang SM, Little SH. Patient-Specific 3-Dimensional Printed Modeling of the Tricuspid Valve for MitraClip Procedure Planning. Circ Cardiovasc Imaging. 2020 Jul;13(7):e010376; *with permission.*)

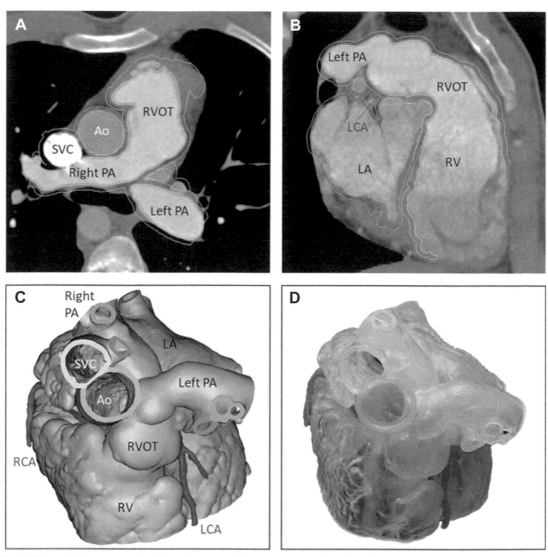

Fig. 4. 3D model in preparation for pulmonary valve intervention. (*A, B*) Cardiac CT imaging was used to create to segment the relevant cardiac structures with a focus on the right heart includes the pulmonary valve and branch pulmonary arteries. (*C*) The digital model represents all the anatomy needed to plan the intervention (*D*) 3D multicolor print based on the digital model. (*From* Pluchinotta FR, Sturla F, Caimi A, Giugno L, Chessa M, Giamberti A, Votta E, Redaelli A, Carminati M. 3-Dimensional personalized planning for transcatheter pulmonary valve implantation in a dysfunctional right ventricular outflow tract. Int J Cardiol. 2020 Jun 15;309:33-39; *with permission.*)

TRANSCATHETER PULMONARY VALVE REPLACEMENT FOR CONGENITAL HEART DISEASE

The right ventricular outflow tract is often reconstructed in patients with conotruncal abnormalities involving the pulmonary valve. For patients with residual lesions such as pulmonary stenosis or pulmonary regurgitation, often seen in tetralogy of Fallot (ToF) for example, further interventions are needed throughout their lives. The right ventricle

can fail in the setting of chronic volume or pressure load from pulmonary valvular dysfunction. To address this, transcatheter pulmonary valve replacements can be used in the appropriate patient with amenable RVOT anatomy. 3D printed models have been found to be useful in the preprocedural planning phase. Pluchinotta and colleagues applied a cardiac CT-based 3D printed model to assess the feasibility of transcatheter pulmonary valve replacement in a 17-year-old male with ToF who had undergone repair with a transannular

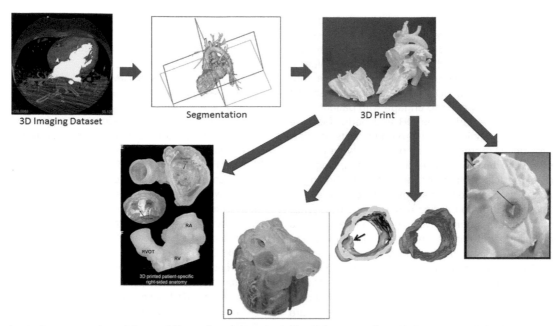

Fig. 5. Representation of the workflow when a 3D print is created, starting from 3D image acquisition to segmentation and then 3D printing. Some of the applications of 3D printing in heart failure included in this review are depicted.

patch in infancy.[24] The patient had severe dilation of the right ventricle and severe pulmonary regurgitation. The aneurysmal nature of the RVOT warranted an advanced imaging technique to assess the potential for a transcatheter approach. Based on the 3D model, it was determined that the proximal and midportions of the RVOT were unfavorable sites for the transcatheter pulmonary valve **(Fig. 4)**. Therefore, the branch pulmonary artery jailing technique was used whereby the right pulmonary artery served as the landing zone for multiple bare-metal stents to anchor the transcatheter pulmonary valve.

TISSUE ENGINEERING/BIOPRINTING

Bioprinting involves the creation of live tissue in a scaffold using cells in the form of bioink. In a study published by Wang and colleagues, they used primary cardiomyocytes isolated from infant rat hearts suspended in a fibrin-based bioink which could then be printed to create cardiac tissue constructs.[25] These cardiac tissue constructs were found to be electromechanically coupled cells that responded as anticipated to known cardiac drugs and continued to develop and mature in vitro. Jang and colleagues found that 3D printed prevascularized stem cell patches using heart tissue-derived extracellular matrix bioink in vivo promoted vascularization and tissue matrix formation.[26] When used in myocardial infarction rat

models, patches also promoted enhanced cardiac function in native tissue as well as neovascularization. In a study conducted by Noor and colleagues, these concepts were taken a step further to create cellularized 3D printed hearts using multiple bioinks.[27] First, they harvested human omental tissue and isolated extracellular matrix and omental cells. The omental tissue cells were then reprogrammed to pluripotent stem cells and differentiated into cardiomyocytes and endothelial cells. Extracellular matrix, cardiomyocytes, and endothelial cells could then be used to form separate biogels used for 3D printing. Using these gels, the authors created patient-specific cardiac patches containing cardiac myocytes and blood vessels modeled after patient CT scans with properties similar to true cardiac tissue. Additionally, in a proof-of-concept model, they used a customized formulation that would support free-form 3D printing of cellular bioink isolated from rats to create small-scale cellularized human hearts with major blood vessels. The potential for the application of bioprinting toward the care of patients with HF continues to be realized.

SUMMARY

3D printing technology has revolutionized personalized medicine, providing patient-specific cardiac models that can be used for education and procedural planning. They serve as noninvasive tools allowing providers to assess complex anatomy in high-risk patients. Treating patients with HF requires precision and planning to optimize outcomes. 3D printing technology is an invaluable tool that can aid in offering these patients personalized care (**Fig. 5**). 3D printed cardiac models can be used by surgeons to engage with patient anatomy before entering the OR and better facilitate operative planning. For interventionalists, models provide 3D representations of anatomy they might otherwise only encounter in 2D. Combining cardiac models with other innovative technologies such as engineering allows investigators to approximate true cardiac tissue properties. While many of the studies involving 3D printed cardiac models include limited numbers of subjects and proof-of-concept methodology secondary to the vast amount of time and detail required to create an accurate patient-specific model, their utility is undeniable and our ability to create them is advancing rapidly. 3D printed cardiac models are important for understanding complex cardiac anatomy and hemodynamics and will undoubtedly become crucial therapeutic tools as well.

CLINICS CARE POINTS

- 3D printing technology should be used to clarify complex spatial cardiac anatomy in patients with HF.
- A high-quality 3D imaging dataset is necessary to produce a high-quality 3D printed model.
- The degree of myocardial resection in patients with HOCM can be planned using a 3D printed cardiac model.
- Preprocedural planning for valve interventions is enhanced using a 3D printed cardiac model.
- 3D models augment other imaging modalities in planning for surgical or transcatheter interventions in patients with CHD.
- Constructs of live cells created via bioprinting may allow cardiac tissue repair in the future.

CONFLICTS OF INTEREST

The authors declare that they have no conflicts of interest to disclose.

REFERENCES

1. Yancy CW, Jessup M, Bozkurt B, et al. ACCF/AHA guideline for the management of heart failure: A report of the American college of cardiology foundation/american heart association task force on practice guidelines. J Am Coll Cardiol 2013;62(16):e147–239.
2. Hollenberg SM, Warner Stevenson L, Ahmad T, et al. ACC expert consensus decision pathway on risk assessment, management, and clinical trajectory of patients hospitalized with heart failure: a report of the American College of Cardiology Solution Set Oversight Committee. J Am Coll Cardiol 2019;74:1966–2011.
3. Tack P, Victor J, Gemmel P, et al. 3D-printing techniques in a medical setting: A systematic literature review. Biomed Eng Online 2016;15(1):115.
4. Andrushchuk U, Adzintsou V, Nevyglas A, et al. Virtual and real septal myectomy using 3-dimensional printed models. Interact Cardiovasc Thorac Surg 2018;26:881–2.
5. Farooqi KM, Gonzalez-Lengua C, Shenoy R, et al. Use of a three dimensional printed cardiac model to assess suitability for biventricular repair. World J Pediatr Congenit Heart Surg 2016;7:414–6.
6. Farooqi KM, Saeed O, Zaidi A, et al. 3D Printing to guide ventricular assist device placement in adults with congenital heart disease and heart failure. JACC Heart Fail 2016;4:301–11.
7. Miller JR, Singh GK, Woodard PK, et al. 3D printing for preoperative planning and surgical simulation of ventricular assist device implantation in a failing systemic right ventricle. J Cardiovasc Comput Tomogr 2020;14:e172–4.
8. Guo HC, Wang Y, Dai J, et al. Application of 3D printing in the surgical planning of hypertrophic obstructive cardiomyopathy and physician-patient communication: A preliminary study. J Thorac Dis 2018;10:867–73.
9. Parachuri VR, Adhyapak SM. The case for surgical myectomy in hypertrophic cardiomyopathy: Is strategic planning the key to success? J Thorac Cardiovasc Surg 2017;154:1687–8.
10. Hermsen JL, Burke TM, Seslar SP, et al. Scan, plan, print, practice, perform: development and use of a patient-specific 3-dimensional printed model in adult cardiac surgery. J Thorac Cardiovasc Surg 2017;153:132–40.
11. Farooqi KM, Mahmood F. Innovations in preoperative planning: insights into another dimension using 3D printing for Cardiac Disease. J Cardiothorac Vasc Anesth 2018;32:1937–45.
12. Biglino G, Capelli C, Wray J, et al. 3D-manufactured patient-specific models of congenital heart defects for communication in clinical practice: feasibility and acceptability. BMJ Open 2015;5(4):e007165.
13. Smerling J, Marboe CC, Lefkowitch JH, et al. Utility of 3D printed cardiac models for medical student education in congenital heart disease: across a spectrum of disease severity. Pediatr Cardiol 2019;40(6):1258–65.

14. Greutmann M, Tobler D, Kovacs AH, et al. Increasing mortality burden among adults with complex congenital heart disease. Congenit Heart Dis 2015;10:117–27.

15. Tuncay V, van Ooijen PMA. 3D printing for heart valve disease: a systematic review. Eur Radiol Exp 2019;3:9.

16. Ripley B, Kelil T, Cheezum MK, et al. 3D printing based on cardiac CT assists anatomic visualization prior to transcatheter aortic valve replacement. J Cardiovasc Comput Tomogr 2016;10:28–36.

17. Qian Z, Wang K, Liu S, et al. Quantitative prediction of paravalvular leak in transcatheter aortic valve replacement based on tissue-mimicking 3D printing. JACC Cardiovasc Imaging 2017;10:719–31.

18. Wang DD, Eng M, Greenbaum A, et al. Predicting LVOT Obstruction After TMVR. JACC Cardiovasc Imaging 2016;9:1349–52.

19. Wang DD, Eng MH, Greenbaum AB, et al. Validating a prediction modeling tool for left ventricular outflow tract (LVOT) obstruction after transcatheter mitral valve replacement (TMVR). Catheter Cardiovasc Interv 2018;92:379–87.

20. Lauten A, Figulla HR, Willich C, et al. Percutaneous caval stent valve implantation: investigation of an interventional approach for treatment of tricuspid regurgitation. Eur Heart J 2010;31(10):1274–81.

21. O'Neill B, Wang DD, Pantelic M, et al. Transcatheter caval valve implantation using multimodality imaging: roles of TEE, CT, and 3D printing. JACC Cardiovasc Imaging 2015;8(2):221–5.

22. Spring AM, Pirelli L, Basman CL, et al. The importance of pre-operative imaging and 3-D printing in transcatheter tricuspid valve-in-valve replacement. Cardiovasc Revasc Med; 2020.

23. Vukicevic M, Faza NN, Avenatti E, et al. Patient-specific 3-Dimensional Printed Modeling of the Tricuspid Valve for MitraClip Procedure Planning. Circ Cardiovasc Imaging 2020;13(7):e010376.

24. Pluchinotta FR, Sturla F, Caimi A, et al. 3-Dimensional personalized planning for transcatheter pulmonary valve implantation in a dysfunctional right ventricular outflow tract. Int J Cardiol 2020;309:33–9.

25. Wang Z, Lee SJ, Cheng HJ, et al. 3D bioprinted functional and contractile cardiac tissue constructs. Acta Biomater 2018;70:48–56.

26. Jang J, Park HJ, Kim SW, et al. 3D printed complex tissue construct using stem cell-laden decellularized extracellular matrix bioinks for cardiac repair. Biomaterials 2017;112:264–74.

27. Noor N, Shapira A, Edri R, et al. 3D printing of personalized thick and perfusable cardiac patches and hearts. Adv Sci (Weinh) 2019;6:1900344.

9780323920193